EASY
HIKES & WALKS
OF SOUTHWESTERN
BRITISH COLUMBIA

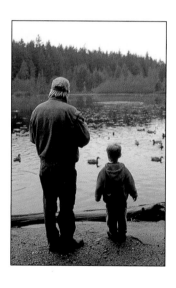

Dawn Hanna

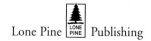

Lone Pine Publishing

The Publisher: Lone Pine Publishing

1901 Raymond Avenue SW, Suite C   10145 – 81 Avenue
Renton, WA, USA 98055   Edmonton, AB, Canada T6E 1W9

Website: www.lonepinepublishing.com

National Library of Canada Cataloguing in Publication Data
Hanna, Dawn, 1959–
    Easy hikes and walks of southwestern British Columbia

    Includes bibliographical references and index.
    ISBN 1-55105-253-9

    1. Hiking—British Columbia—Lower Mainland—Guidebooks. 2. Walking—British Columbia—Lower Mainland—Guidebooks. 3. Trails—British Columbia—Lower Mainland—Guidebooks. 4. Lower Mainland (B.C.)—Guidebooks. I. Title.
GV199.44.C22L68 2002   917.11'3044   C2002-910558-7

Editorial Director: Nancy Foulds
Illustrations Coordinator: Carol Woo
Production Coordinator: Jennifer Fafard
Book Design: Rod Michalchuk
Layout & Production: Monica Triska
Map Work: Volker Bodegom
Cover Design: Rod Michalchuk
Scanning, Separations & Film: Elite Lithographers Co.

Cover photo: PhotoDisc, Image Ideas Inc./PictureQuest
All other photos by Dawn Hanna

The following people have illustrations on the designated page numbers: Gary Ross: 14, 16, 24, 26, 34, 52, 69, 98, 106, 145, 148, 152, 156, 158, 165, 166, 175, 183, 214, 219, 223, 225, 232; Ian Sheldon: 66, 93, 97, 162, 210, 229; Linda Kershaw: 79; Ted Nordhagen: 134, 196, 200.

We acknowledge the financial support of the Government of Canada through the Book Publishing Industry Development Program (BPIDP) for our publishing activities.

PC: P4

Contents

Preface

The first time my feet ever trod a trail, I was a kid. I can still remember marvelling at the tallness of the trees, the sweetness of the huckleberries and the noisy riffles of the Capilano River. It was a different world from the streets, alleys and beaches of Kitsilano that I was used to exploring.

Years later, I realize that those early hiking experiences were more than just field trips. In fact, they opened my eyes to the natural world and its wonders.

Back then, people were more mesmerized by the plants, animals and landscapes of exotic lands than by nature nearby. It was the era of *Wild Kingdom*, in which Marlin Perkins and his trusty sidekick, Jim, tracked lions, rhinos and crocodiles—not tree frogs, Douglas's squirrels and water striders. So, like many kids, I ended up knowing more about the natural wonders of far-flung places than I did about the plants and animals in my own backyard.

As an adult, though, I learned more about the inhabitants of the forests, lakes and rivers closer to home. I learned more about the relationships between plants and animals—and how they are affected by people. And I learned about the problems facing some of those plants and animals: habitat loss, pollution and competition from introduced species.

As I became informed, I wanted to do something to ensure that the plants and animals I had grown up with would still be there in the future. That desire got me thinking that if more people knew more about the wild wonders of BC and the problems that face them, then maybe more people would work to find solutions.

Now that I am a mom, my desire to keep BC wild and wondrous is even stronger. I want my son to have the chance to hear the scolding chatter of a Douglas's squirrel, to see thousand-year-old trees and to smell the unforgettable stench of a spawned-out salmon. I want him to thrill at the sight of an osprey's nest perched high on a river piling, to explore the miniature world of a moss garden and to imagine the vast sheets of ice that scoured the Lower Mainland thousands of years ago.

In essence, I want my treasure to have the opportunity to know the other treasures we share the planet with.

For Sam

As long as you live, hear the waterfalls and birds and winds sing. Interpret the rocks, learn the language of flood, storm and the avalanche. Acquaint yourself with glaciers and wild gardens, and get as near the heart of the world as you can.

— from the words of John Muir

Introduction

Even seasoned backpackers sometimes want an easy hike that can be
completed at a relaxed pace. Maybe
you've had a long, tiring week, but
you still want to get some fresh air
and gentle exercise. Maybe you want
to hike with someone who has
reduced mobility. Maybe you belong
to a group of active seniors who
meet weekly for a short, scenic outing in the great outdoors.

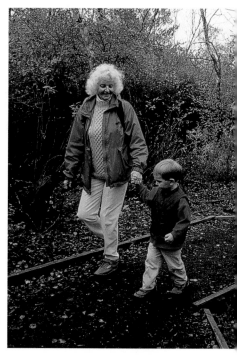

Or maybe you want to take a baby
or young kids along. And, as any par-
ent knows, going on a hike with kids
is a whole different adventure from
going on a hike with other adults.
Children don't have the same physical stamina or attention span as most
adults, and they need shorter outings. Sure, you might be able to do
Mount Seymour in a five-hour return hike, but at what cost? Tired,
cranky kids? Even more tired, more cranky adults?

That said, there are definite advantages to hiking with children. For one
thing, you'll see things through different eyes—eyes that can find treasures among the dirt and rocks, imaginary animals among the foliage and
a whole new world in the muddy trickle of a tiny creek. If you hike with
children, be prepared to see things in a whole new light, even along trails
you may have walked hundreds of times before.

Disclaimer

Hiking, like all outdoor activities, involves an element of the unknown
and thus, an element of risk. Weather, erosion and other forces may
change the conditions or route of a trail. Therefore, keep in mind that
this book serves as a guide only. It is the ultimate and sole responsibility of the readers to determine which hikes are appropriate to their skills
or fitness levels and those of their party. Hikers also hold the ultimate
and sole responsibility to be aware of and alert to any changes or hazards that might have occurred since the research and writing of this
book.

Overview Map

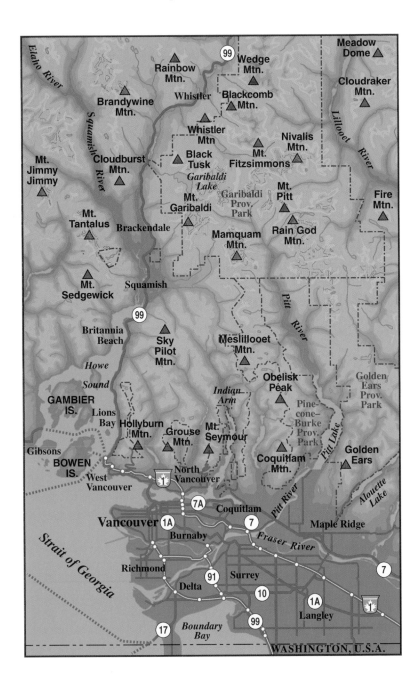

About the Hike Descriptions

The outings described in this guide are organized by area, beginning with those in and close to Vancouver. At the back of the book you'll find an alphabetical index, as well as lists to help you choose a destination according to the hike's duration, season or difficulty.

Distance & Time

All distances indicated for hikes are for *return* trips. The corresponding times given are approximate; take into account your group's hiking style. A group of quick hikers who make only brief stops to check out a hike's particular features will cover a few kilometres much faster than sauntering hikers who linger along the way. And be sure to allow more than enough time to return before the daylight fades.

Maps

The maps that accompany the hikes in this book are meant to indicate the general location and direction of each trail; they are not navigational aids. Park maps and topographical maps provide more detail (see 'Information Sources,' p. 248).

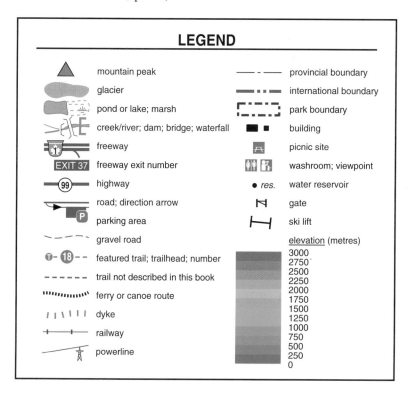

LEGEND

mountain peak		provincial boundary	
glacier		international boundary	
pond or lake; marsh		park boundary	
creek/river; dam; bridge; waterfall		building	
freeway		picnic site	
freeway exit number		washroom; viewpoint	
highway		water reservoir	
road; direction arrow		gate	
parking area		ski lift	
gravel road		elevation (metres)	
featured trail; trailhead; number		3000 2750 2500 2250 2000 1750 1500 1250 1000 750 500 250 0	
trail not described in this book			
ferry or canoe route			
dyke			
railway			
powerline			

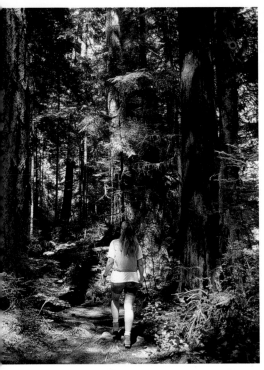

Ratings

Although most adults will consider the hikes in this book quite easy, remember that the ratings are geared to kids.

Easy hikes can be done by children of almost any age; they are generally flat and short.

Moderate hikes involve more rugged terrain with a few ups and downs along the way. Younger kids will have to work harder, but older kids shouldn't have any problems.

Tough hikes, because of their steepness or uneven ground, are best left to older kids. Younger kids could do these trips, but only if they're experienced hikers or if there's an adult willing to provide a piggyback ride if necessary.

Access & Driving Time

Unless otherwise stated, the access description assumes that you are coming from the Vancouver city centre. The estimated driving time assumes good driving conditions. Allow more time during peak traffic periods.

With the following two exceptions, all trailheads are accessible by two-wheel-drive vehicles: for Cougar Mountain, a two-wheel-drive vehicle will bring you within a kilometre of the trailhead; for Widgeon Falls, the water access requires a canoe or kayak.

Trailheads

Every hike starts at a trailhead. The most helpful ones have signs and maps. Others, such as Cougar Mountain and Iona Beach, don't have any signs at the trailheads, but their starting points should still be obvious.

Unfortunately, trailheads often attract thieves as well as hikers. To make your vehicle a less tempting target, leave nothing inside. If your vehicle is broken into, report it to the local police or RCMP. The police may not be able to recover any stolen goods, but your report may result in an increased police presence and fewer break-ins in the future.

Equipment & Other Essentials

Wearing the right gear and carrying the essentials are important for any hiker. When you hike with kids, it's even more critical to be properly equipped—you're responsible for more than just your own safety and well-being. Here's a look at some of the stuff you'll need.

Clothing & Footwear

The hikes and walks in this book cover many different kinds of terrain. Some sections of trail are groomed and gravelled, whereas others may be muddy or have roots and rocks poking up. The weather is another variable: some days may start off warm but cool off when the clouds move in; other days may start off in drizzle but break into toasty sunshine. Fortunately, there are ways to dress that will keep you prepared but prevent you from having to lug along a dresserful of clothes.

The best way to dress is in layers. For warm weather, start with shorts and a T-shirt. Nylon shorts are best because if they get wet the fabric will dry more quickly than cotton and lessen the chances of your getting chilled if the temperature drops. (Even if the sun is shining, it can feel much cooler high in the mountains, in the shade of the forest or in the wind.)

A cotton T-shirt is fine in summer, but it's best to carry a spare in case the first gets soaked. (Again, wet cotton will suck warmth from a body.) Also take along a light fleece or wool sweater so that if it does cool down, you've got an extra layer for warmth. Windproof nylon pants are also good to pack, and lightweight. Leave the jeans at home. They're heavy, and if they get wet they'll not only chill you, they'll get heavier.

For cool or wet weather in fall, winter and spring—and sometimes summer—make the first (inner) layer polyester or polypropylene. Although some people spend big bucks on international name brands, proper clothing doesn't have to be expensive. Places such as Mountain Equipment Co-op offer good-quality polyester tops and bottoms at much lower prices, especially for kids. The second cool-weather layer should be lightweight fleece or wool. Again, the price varies with the brand name. The last layer should be waterproof and can be a one-piece rainsuit, a rain poncho, or a combination of rain pants and a rainjacket. If you're shopping for kids, bear in mind that separate pieces accommodate a child's growth spurts better than one-piece suits. An umbrella may be useful on some hikes, particularly if your child backpack has no canopy.

Most walks and hikes in this book can be done with a sturdy pair of running shoes. Hiking shoes or boots provide additional stability and protection on rocky, rooty, sometimes slippery terrain. If hikes are going to be a regular part of your weekend activities, it's worth investing in good boots.

Finally, consider your socks. Most experienced hikers wear an inner sock of very light polypropylene that can wick moisture away from the skin to an outer sock of polyester or wool. Avoid cotton socks, period. Cotton absorbs sweat and provides the perfect conditions for blisters.

Keep a change of clothes—including socks and shoes—waiting in the vehicle (in the trunk, out of sight of thieves, of course) for each person for after the hike. That way, if it's wet, muddy or cold on the trail, you can all slip into clean, dry clothes and be more comfortable for the ride home.

Food & Drink

Even if you're just going walking for an hour or two, bring along fluids and a little snack. Water and unsweetened juice, fruit (dried or fresh), granola bars, fig bars, carrot sticks, cheese and crackers are good choices.

If you're out for a longer hike, pack a lunch that includes sandwiches, some fruit or vegetables and a few energy-rich extras, such as raisins, dried apricots, granola bars and fig bars.

Always take plenty of water for the time that you will be hiking as well as for lunchtime. Never assume water will be available along your hike.

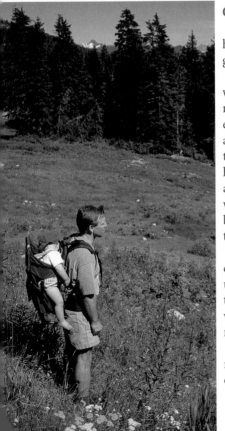

Carriers & Backpacks

If your child is too small to hike on his or her own, you'll need to invest in a good carrier or backpack.

A carrier can be a great, lightweight way to transport a baby under six months of age. Look for a carrier that is easy to put on, is easy to adjust and allows a baby to be carried facing toward or away from you. It should have ample padding at the shoulders and hips, and distribute the baby's weight in a way that won't leave you bowed over and aching at the end of the trip.

A child backpack is usually a more comfortable way to carry a baby, but using a backpack is not a good idea until the baby can hold his or her head up well. Most manufacturers recommend a minimum age of six months.

Child backpacks come in a variety of makes and models. The most expensive one is not necessarily the best—you

should choose the backpack that best fits you and your baby. Here are some basic features you should look for:
- lots of padding on the hip belt and shoulder straps
- an adjustable fit for adults of different heights
- an adjustable safety harness for the baby
- a storage compartment big enough to hold diapers, wipes, food and other baby paraphernalia
- a support stand that allows the backpack to stand on its own. (Never leave a baby in a backpack supported by only its stand, because the slightest movement can tip both over in an instant.)

Try to get as light a child backpack as possible, because you're going to have to carry not just the backpack but also your baby and all the baby gear. Before making a purchase, be sure to try the backpack on with weight in it.

If you're buying used, be sure to research which backpacks have had safety recalls (see 'Information Sources', p. 249).

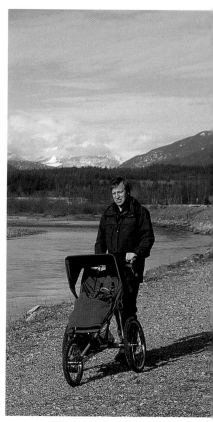

Strollers & All-Terrain Strollers

Some stroller models are fairly rugged. If you have a stroller with large wheels and good rubber treads, you can probably navigate the bumps and lumps of many dirt or gravel paths.

If you plan to attempt more rugged hiking trails, with their inevitable roots, rocks, drops and mud puddles, you'll need something more trail-friendly: an all-terrain stroller (also known as a jogging stroller). All-terrain strollers are not recommended for babies younger than six months, and avoid really bumpy trails until the baby is at least one year old, because all that bumping and jarring could damage a baby's tender brain.

When all-terrain strollers first came on the market, there were only a few brands available. These days there are many to choose from. A word of caution: you get what you pay for. Yes, unfortunately, the $100 discount-store model is not as well made as the $400 model, nor does it have as many great features. My advice is to invest in the better model. It will last longer and function better. With luck, you may be able to find one second-hand.

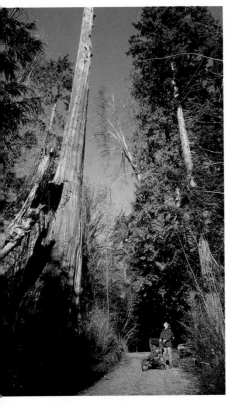

We bit the bullet and bought one that has 46-centimetre (18-inch) wheels, an adjustable seat and a rain cover. It folds up nicely to go in the car and is remarkably lightweight. Whether you buy a top-of-the-line model or a less expensive version, look for these features:

- a wrist strap to prevent the stroller from rolling out of reach if you lose your grip
- a deep seat to keep the baby from moving from side to side
- a restraining belt, crotch strap and, if possible, shoulder straps to secure the baby
- a hand brake to slow the stroller quickly
- air-filled wheels, 41 centimetres (16 inches) in diameter or larger, for optimum shock absorption. (If you're on a particularly bumpy trail, deflate the tires a bit for better shock absorption.)

Other Essentials

1. Guidebook or map or both. If you're going for a two-hour outing along Boundary Bay, it's a pretty safe bet that you won't get lost. But in other places, such as the forests and mountains of the North Shore or even the forests of Stanley Park and Pacific Spirit Regional Park, it can be surprisingly easy to find yourself off-track. A good guidebook will help you avoid such unplanned adventures. It's also a good idea to take along a detailed map of the area.

2. Sunscreen, sunglasses and hat. The sunscreen should be SPF 15 or better. The sunglasses should screen both UVA and UVB rays. The hat should have a brim to shield the face, the eyes and, if possible, the neck from the sun or rain.

3. First-aid kit. The first-aid kit should contain the basics: bandages, gauze, adhesive tape, antiseptic towelettes, an elastic tensor bandage, pain reliever (both adult and children's), tweezers, moleskin for blisters and a small pair of scissors. Pack along an orange garbage bag as well, for an instant rain poncho, pack cover or emergency overnight shelter if you get lost or stranded.

4. Pocket knife. Infinitely useful. Once you have one, you'll wonder how you ever lived without it.

5. Flashlight or headlamp. Even if you allowed for lots of time to return before dark, unforeseen events may delay you. A flashlight or headlamp will help to light the way and illuminate whatever you're fumbling with in the dark, be it map, first-aid supplies or pocket knife.

Trail Ethics

Stay on the trail. Trails create easier access into an area, and they protect that area from mass trampling and the destruction that results. Resist the temptation to take erosion-causing shortcuts on switchbacks, and always use constructed stairs. Don't trample subalpine meadows just to avoid a mud puddle or two.

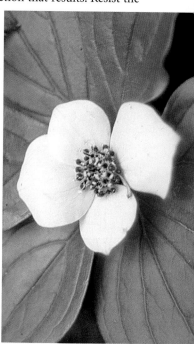

Pack out all your garbage. Do not leave behind anything that you brought with you. Garbage is not only an unpleasant sight for the next hiker, but it attracts animals that can be nuisances or hazards.

Don't pick any wildflowers or other plants. Don't dig up shrubs or carry off rocks or any items with heritage significance. In essence, don't take anything with you that you didn't bring in. Follow the famous hiker's credo: Take only photographs, leave only footprints.

If you hike with young children, you'll have to wait until they're older for them to understand the importance of following these ethics. The best way to encourage respect for the trails and the environment is to set a good example.

Peeing in the Woods

Sometimes you're on a trail and you just have to go. Maybe there are no toilets nearby, maybe you just can't make it in time. Be prepared for these situations and carry a small roll of toilet paper or a pocket pack of tissues and a couple of plastic bags.

The basic rule is to do your business at least 45 metres (150 feet) from any stream, lake or other body of water. If you're dealing with poop, dig a shallow hole in the soil beforehand and bury your deposit after. Pack used toilet paper in a plastic bag and carry it out with your garbage.

Encounters with Wildlife

Flying Bugs

These critters are the wildlife you're most likely to encounter on the trail. In summer, mosquitoes, no-see-ums, blackflies and deerflies can ruin an otherwise lovely day hike. Your best defence is bug spray, though bug-proof clothing can help. Some people swear by insect repellents that contain DEET (also known as N, N-diethyl-metatoluamide), but be aware that this stuff is potent enough to dissolve plastic, paint and some synthetic fabrics.

Ticks

Ticks are most worrisome in April through June, but remember that ticks can be around at any time of the year. Although you won't find them on most of the hikes and walks in this book, there are some areas (such as West and North Vancouver and Bowen Island) where ticks can show up even in backyards. Wearing long pants tucked into socks is a good way to fend off ticks.

These little sesame seed–sized creatures can latch on when you are walking along a brush-lined trail. They then look for some warm and furry part into which to sink their pincer-like jaws. Therefore, you'll need to check closely—especially such parts as armpits, groin, head and back—after each walk or hike. Use your fingers as well as your eyes to find any unusual bumps on the skin. Ticks can be the size of a pinhead, so check carefully.

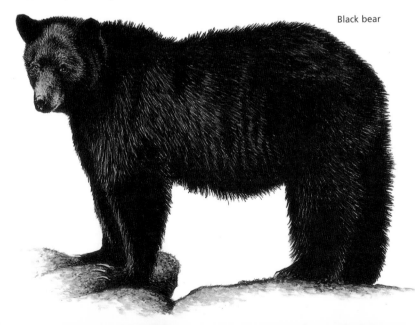

Black bear

If you do find a tick embedded in the skin, resist the initial impulse to rip it out. A tick must be removed carefully. If its body is crushed while you're trying to remove it, the contents of its gut, along with any insidious bacteria that it may contain, can be transferred into your blood.

It's best to have a doctor remove the tick as soon as possible. If that's not feasible, you can do it yourself using tick pliers. Grasp the tick close to the skin and gently pull it straight out, taking care not to squish it. Do not apply petroleum jelly, alcohol or a hot match to make the tick back out; these methods do not work and will only increase the risk of disease transmission. Put the tick into a plastic bag or a vial with some damp cotton or grass and make sure that it goes to the Centre for Disease Control laboratories for testing.

Even if you successfully remove the tick yourself, you should see a doctor at the earliest opportunity. These days, it's standard for anyone who has been bitten by a tick to start on a program of antibiotics, just in case the tick was carrying *Borrelia burgdorferi* bacteria, which are responsible for Lyme disease. Although Lyme disease won't kill you, it is imperative that it be treated as soon as possible. Left untreated, Lyme disease can be debilitating and painful.

Bears

Your chances of seeing a bear on most of the trails described in this book are very small. Bears have been known to show up along popular trails in West Vancouver, North Vancouver, Port Coquitlam and Maple Ridge, so it's best to know how to react should you encounter one.

If you do come upon a bear, most likely it will be a black bear. Grizzly bears live as far south as Whistler, but they tend to avoid people.

In the Lower Mainland, black bears have adapted to the presence of people. They may appear quite harmless, but they are very definitely wild animals, and, as such, are quite capable of harming you.

It is true that these powerful animals have seriously injured and killed people, but such attacks are extremely rare. In BC, between 1963 and 1992, bears fatally mauled 12 people. In the past 10 years, bears have injured about 25 people in the province. You can help keep those numbers down by learning more about bears and by practising bear-aware strategies on the trail.

Make noise. To let the bear know that you are approaching and to give it time to leave the area, talk loudly, sing, shout or clap your hands. Forget about using 'bear-bells' (small bells attached to your pack or clothing while you hike). 'In Glacier National Park,' says BC Wildlife Branch bear biologist Tony Hamilton, 'it's like ringing a dinner bell. The bears there have clued in that the bells mean food is coming. The sound of the human voice is far better.'

Keep your distance. Never approach a bear. If you're too close for a bear's comfort, it may consider you a threat and act accordingly. Even if you see a cub apparently on its own, no matter how cute it is, stay away, because the protective mother is sure to be close at hand. And *never*—as some witless parents have been known to do—tell your child to move closer to a bear, or to any other wild animal, so that you can take a photo.

Never try to feed a bear. Not only is it dangerous for you, but a bear with a taste for human food often ends up dead.

Don't hike with dogs. Dogs can antagonize bears, sometimes bringing on an attack. An unleashed dog may also lead a bear back to you.

Back away. If you do come upon a bear, you can minimize how threatening you appear by backing away slowly while waving your arms slowly and talking in a calm voice (to help the bear recognize you as human). *Never* turn and run, because the bear might chase after you.

Cougars

Although it's extremely rare to see cougars on the trail, it does happen. In recent years, for example, cougars have been seen in the Seymour Demonstration Forest in North Vancouver. Children are more likely than adults to be the target of a cougar attack, but at least two incidents in BC in the past few years have involved adults.

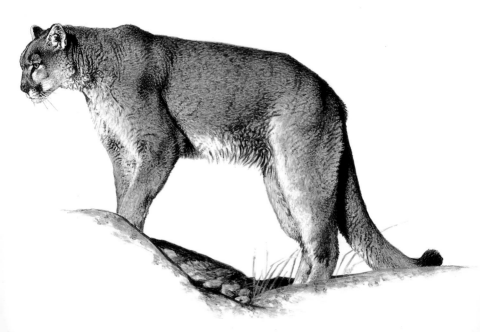

Tell Somebody

Be sure to let someone dependable know where you're going and when to expect you back. If you're heading out for a hike some distance from home, include details such as what you're wearing, what vehicle you're using to get there and who's going with you.

As with bears, your best defence is to make noise on the trail. Use your voice—sing or speak loudly. Given half a chance, most cougars will avoid people.

Make sure that children are always within your direct view, especially when hiking in places where cougars have been seen.

If you do encounter a cougar, pick up any small children immediately. Children frighten easily, and their quick movements can provoke an attack. It's also recommended that you make yourself look as big and bad as you possibly can—wave your arms and make a lot of noise, all the time backing up slowly. *Never* turn and run, because it may trigger the animal's innate predatory response.

If the cougar approaches, throw rocks or sticks or whatever is on hand. Again, you want to impress upon the cougar that you will not be an easy meal.

Kid Safety

In a perfect world, every child would walk one metre ahead of the adults and never wander. In the real world, however, toddlers may choose to play hide-and-seek in the middle of the forest, and older kids may be lured off the trail by a bounding squirrel. Kids of all ages may decide to do a little off-road adventuring on their own, without telling Mom or Dad.

For these reasons, it's a good idea to plan on your children getting lost. You want to make sure that both you and the kids have some strategies to deal with such a situation.

- Teach your kids the importance of staying on the trail at all times.
- Dress kids in bright colours that stand out against forest vegetation.
- Tie bells to their shoes—the tinkling sounds can help you keep track of kids during those seconds when you turn your head and they wander away.
- Attach whistles to jacket zippers or safety-pin them to shirts. Teach the children that if they get separated from you they should blow three times, wait, and then do it over and over again until you find them.
- Allow kids six and older to carry their own backpacks with some essentials (water, snacks, plastic garbage bag, jacket, hat).
- As soon as they can understand, teach children the basics of the Hug-a-Tree Program.

The Hug-a-Tree Program

In 1981, three brothers aged 7, 9 and 15 went for a hike only a kilometre away from their campsite in a state park in California. Deciding to take a shortcut, the nine-year-old became separated from his brothers. He failed to return to the campsite. After four days of searching, rescuers found the boy's body about 4 kilometres from the campground. He had died of hypothermia.

Shortly afterward, the Hug-a-Tree and Survive Program (its full name) was developed. Its aim is to teach kids a few basic principles for staying safe in the wilderness.

Below is a summary of those ideas, courtesy of the Provincial Emergency Program. Teach them to your kids.

Always tell someone where you are going. That way, if you do get lost, searchers will know where to start looking.

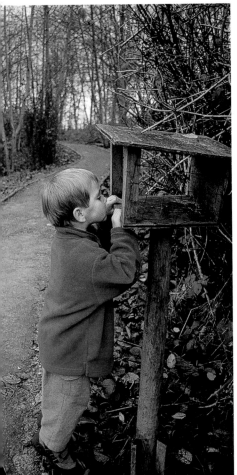

Always carry a bright orange garbage bag and a whistle. Make a hole in the bag big enough for your face, then put the bag over your head. It will help keep you dry and warm. You can blow the whistle to let people know where you are. It will carry farther than your voice.

Admit to yourself when you get lost. Anyone can get lost, adults or kids. Don't feel bad about getting lost. And don't worry that you'll get in trouble. Your parents will be very happy to see you. When you are lost, you need to use your head to help yourself.

Hug a tree. When you know you're lost, it can be frightening to be alone. Hugging a tree and even talking to it will help calm you down and prevent you from panicking. By staying in one place you'll be easier to find than if you keep moving around, and you won't accidentally wander farther from help.

Help the searchers find you. If you hear people yelling and whistling, answer them. Yell back or blow your whistle. Searchers are your friends—many of them are moms and dads themselves—and they're trying to find you and help you get back home. (Some lost kids have tried to hide from searchers because they were afraid.)

Make yourself big. If you hear a helicopter overhead, get out into the open and wave your orange garbage bag. If you can, use rocks or sticks or even drag your foot in the ground to make a big S.O.S. sign.

Make noise. If you hear an animal noise, yell at it—if it's a wild animal, it will run away, but, if it's a search dog looking for you, your shouting will help the search party find you.

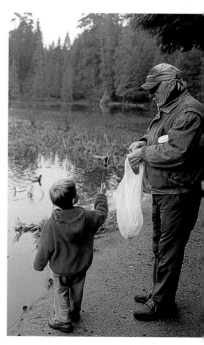

Don't run. Never run from a wild animal; make noise instead. And don't run around if you are lost; it is much better to stay in one place until somebody finds you. (Fears of the dark and 'of lions and tigers and bears' are a big factor in panicking children into running. They need strong reassurance to stay put and be safe.)

Hug-a-Tree also recommends that parents footprint their children before starting out to help searchers in the event a child gets lost. To make the print, put a piece of aluminum foil on a soft surface, such as a rug or a folded towel. Have your child walk across the foil—with whatever boots or shoes he or she will wear when hiking. Then mark the foil with the child's name and put it in a safe place. This print will help trackers distinguish your child's footprint from others in the area and help them to find him or her more quickly.

With some planning and the right precautions in place, you'll just have one thing to remember on your walk or hike, and that's to have fun!

Stanley Park

Length: 4-km loop

Time needed: 2 to 2.5 hours

Season: Year-round

Rating: Easy

Dogs: Yes, on leash

Stroller-friendly: All-terrain strollers only

Washrooms: At Third Beach

Highlights: Western redcedar, skid roads, Beaver Lake, candelabra trees, Eastern grey and Douglas's squirrels

Access: Take Georgia Street westbound to Stanley Park. Turn right and follow park drive around to Third Beach and park in pay lot.

Driving time: 15 minutes

Every day, whether it's sunny, raining or snowing, lots of people walk Stanley Park's seawall, but they often forget about the many kilometres of trails that criss-cross the interior of the park. Here you can see huge old-growth trees, look for tiny songbirds and stroll around water-lilied lakes.

Start at the parking area and walk toward the huge bigleaf maple tree. Where three trails diverge, take the middle path and follow the signs toward Prospect Point and the Hollow Tree. A few minutes of uphill walking will bring you to another big tree—a huge western redcedar tree, which, at almost 40 metres tall and 14 metres around, is the largest western redcedar in the park.

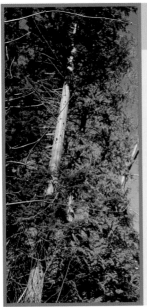

Western Redcedar
(Thuja plicata)

Stanley Park's biggest western redcedar stands about 40 metres high and almost 14 metres around. It once stood five metres taller, but its top has been lopped off. In the 1960s, the parks board considered that it posed a risk of falling. The tree is now about the same size as the Point Atkinson Lighthouse (see p. 78).

An even bigger western redcedar grows near Cheewhat Lake on Vancouver Island. That cedar stands 59 metres tall and measures almost 19 metres around. It's hard to imagine how big this tree is without seeing it, but imagine if you stacked 30 men one on top of the other—that'd be about how tall the redcedar is. If you had 10 men stretch out their arms and form a circle, that'd be about how wide around the redcedar is.

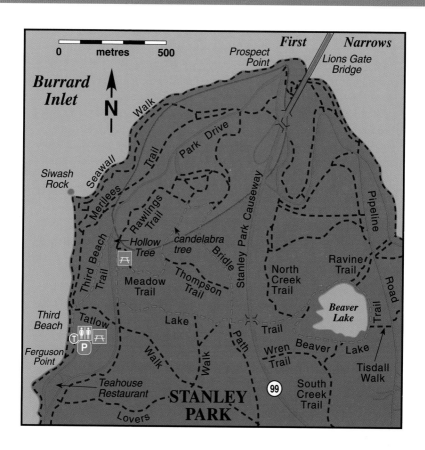

0 metres 500

Burrard Inlet

N

First Narrows

Prospect Point

Lions Gate Bridge

Siwash Rock

Seawall

Merilees

Rawlings Trail

Hollow Tree

candelabra tree

Bridle

Stanley Park Causeway

Pipeline

Third Beach Trail

Meadow Trail

Thompson Trail

North Creek Trail

Ravine Trail

Road

Third Beach

Tatlow

Lake

Path

Beaver Lake

Trail

Ferguson Point

Walk

Walk

Wren Trail

Beaver Lake

Tisdall Walk

Teahouse Restaurant

STANLEY PARK

99

South Creek Trail

Lovers

Park Drive

Walk

Trail

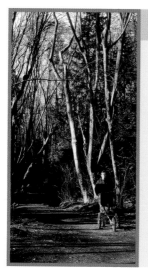

Skid Roads

A skid road is a path that loggers used to drag cut trees out of the forest. Because it's difficult to drag trees over muddy ground, these paths were built, and planks or slabs of wood were laid across them. Sometimes oil was brushed onto the wood to make the logs skid even better.

From the 1860s until the 1880s, five logging companies were cutting the trees in what is now Stanley Park. Not all of the park has been logged. You can usually tell which parts were logged by the presence of old tree stumps and the absence of really big trees. Compare the size of the trees on the first part of the hike (they're all hemlocks) to the older trees you'll see later.

Once past the redcedar tree, continue uphill to reach the roadway. Cross it and take a look at the Hollow Tree. It once measured 18.3 metres around, but now it's actually more of a hollow stump. It serves as a 'nurse log' to smaller trees that grow from its nooks and crannies.

Cross the meadow, heading south by southeast, and look for a big, wide-open bark-mulch trail, called the Meadow Trail. About 130 years ago, before it was a trail, it was a skid road. If you look closely as you walk the Meadow Trail, you can still see some old skid planks buried in the ground.

Turn left at the first intersection on the trail. About 100 metres farther on stand some big western redcedar trees, including one that splits about halfway up. These trees with two or more tops are called 'candelabra trees,' because the tops look like the arms of a candelabra (see p. 23).

At the next intersection, go right. A bit farther ahead, at the next intersection, go right again to join onto the Bridle Path Trail. As you head downhill, traffic noise filters in from the causeway. Pass the little wooden shelter, and walk a bit farther to the next intersection. Go left over the overpass.

Follow the paved path into the forest. The path becomes gravel. At the fork in the path, go right onto the Lake Trail. Continue straight ahead through the next intersection. Beaver Lake can be seen on the left through the trees. The First Nations people who used to live near what is now Lumberman's Arch called Beaver Lake *Ahka-Chu*, meaning 'little lake.'

At the next fork, stay left to continue along the shore. Benches along this section are a good place to stop to have a snack or watch the resident ducks and other birds. You might also see some other familiar park animals, such as squirrels (see p. 23).

Beaver Lake

Many years ago the Lake Trail path was right on the shoreline of Beaver Lake. The lake has shrunk over the years: in 1938 the lake measured almost 7 hectares in size, but now it covers only about 4 hectares.

The phenomenon responsible for the shrinking of the lake is called 'meadow lake formation.' In simple terms, it begins when the aquatic plants in the water decay. This process takes oxygen out of the lake. The dead plant matter builds up, the lake becomes shallower, and other plants begin to grow on the lake edges.

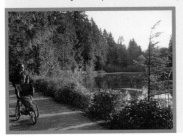

Unless the lake is dredged to remove some of the dead plant material and mud, the lake will become a marsh, then a meadow. Eventually, the area formerly under water will become forested.

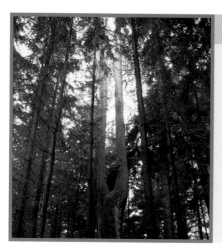

Candelabra Trees

Why do 'candelabra trees' grow this strange way? A candelabra tree starts off growing normally—straight up and with one top—but then the tree goes through a drought or a period when not many nutrients are reaching its roots, so it dies back a bit. When water and nutrients are once again available, the tree sends up a new top, and it then has two or possibly more tops.

Continue around the lake until you return to the Lake Trail. Retrace your steps over the overpass. Take the trail straight ahead. You will reach an intersection. Stay right to continue on the Lake Trail. Walk straight ahead until, about 15 to 20 minutes later, you come to a T junction. Go right on the Rawlings Trail to return to the meadow and the Hollow Tree. Then retrace your steps across the roadway, past the huge redcedar and back to Third Beach.

Eastern Grey Squirrel *(Sciurus carolinensis)* & Douglas's Squirrel *(Tamiasciurus douglasi)*

Two kinds of squirrels are found in Stanley Park: Douglas's squirrels, which are native to southwestern BC, and grey squirrels, which are not. Remarkably, all the grey squirrels that you see in Stanley Park and everywhere else in Greater Vancouver are descended from three or four pairs of eastern grey squirrels that were let loose in the park around 1914.

Despite its name, the eastern grey squirrel can be grey or black. It eats leaf buds, leaves, fruits, seeds and nuts—the same kinds of things that the Douglas's squirrel eats—and it builds its nests in holes in dead trees—just like the Douglas's squirrel does. But grey squirrels are bigger than Douglas's squirrels and are more aggressive. Therefore, in places where both squirrel species are found, the Douglas's squirrel has to compete with a bigger, tougher opponent for food and shelter.

The grey squirrel also has another advantage: female greys can give birth to two litters of baby squirrels each year, whereas female Douglas's squirrels can have only one litter each year.

Jericho Park

Length: 3-km loop

Time needed: 1.5 to 2 hours

Season: Year-round

Rating: Easy

Dogs: Yes, on leash

Stroller-friendly: Yes

Washrooms: Near parking lot at beginning of hike

Highlights: Red-winged black-birds, rabbits, large-leaved lupine, cattails

Access: Follow Vancouver's Point Grey Road to its westernmost end. Park in lot. Note: Pay parking from May to October.

Driving time: 20 minutes

Start from the southwest corner of the parking lot and follow the wide gravel path westward as it winds along the shore of a small pond, then into the open woods. In a few minutes, you will arrive at a larger pond where you can enjoy many different bird calls and bird songs.

At the end of the pond, where the path comes to a junction, go right and follow an old road as it curves westward along a shallow marshy area. Barn swallows, cliff swallows and other small birds flit around here. You may also see dragonflies. And, a little farther, near the blackberry bushes, you might also see some rabbits. These rabbits are not native to the park.

Where the road meets the next path, go left onto the gravel. Cross a small bridge over a tiny creek and follow this path to arrive back at the big pond. Go right up the bark-mulch path for a good view of the park and the sea. Then, at the first pathway, go right again. During spring and summer, many varieties of purply blue lupines grow on both sides of the path.

Rabbits

The rabbits that you see in Jericho Park come in many sizes and colours. Some of them are very shy while others might eat a lettuce leaf or blades of grass right from your hand. All of the rabbits in the park were once someone's pet or were born to someone's pet. Their owners bought them as

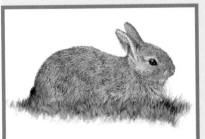

babies, but later released them into the park—a bad idea, because rabbits from a pet store are not meant to live in the wild. They can get diseases, or they might be eaten by coyotes. Before getting a rabbit for a pet, make sure that you are prepared to give it a good home for its entire life.

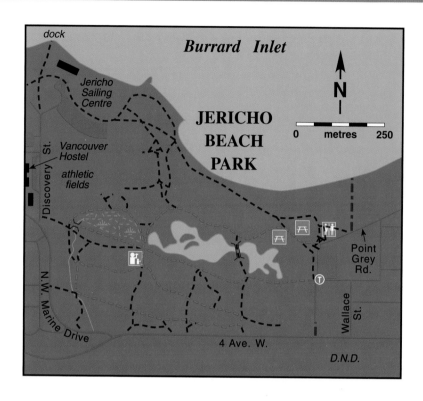

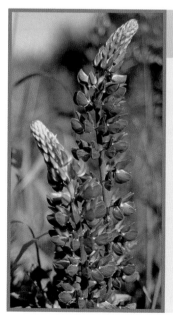

Large-leaved Lupine
(Lupinus polyphyllus)

The large-leaved lupine is just one of the many different species of lupine that grow in BC. Most lupines have bluish to purplish flowers, but some have pink or yellow flowers.

The lupines belong to the same plant family (Leguminosae or Fabaceae) as peas, beans, peanuts and soybeans. Some species, such as the Nootka lupine, are a favourite food of bears. Others, such as seashore lupine, were eaten by First Nations people. Look closely at the lupines here, and you may see what look like hairy pea-pods about as big as a child's finger. Inside are tiny 'peas' or seeds. Don't eat them, because some lupine seeds are **poisonous.**

Red-winged Blackbird *(Agelaius phoeniceus)*

In southwestern BC you will often hear the *konk-a-ree* of the red-winged blackbird. Male red-winged blackbirds are about the same size as starlings, but they are all black with bright red or reddish-orange shoulder patches, called epaulettes. Female red-winged blackbirds, however, are a mottled brown with just a bit of orange on their shoulders.

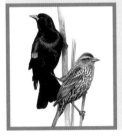

Most of the year you can see red-winged blackbirds among the cattails in the pond in Jericho Park. In springtime, each male red-wing chases off other males from the part of the marsh that he has staked out as his own. When a male wants to chase away a competitor, his puffs up the red patches on his shoulders, like a weightlifter flexing his muscles. A male also puffs up his shoulders when a female comes by.

Jericho Park views

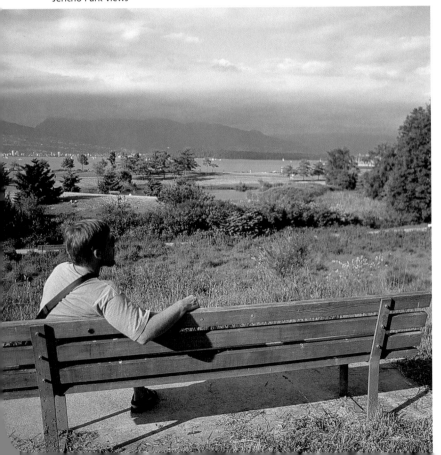

Continue along to a fork in the path and go left onto an old road. In summer, walking on this road can feel as if you're walking through a long, green tunnel because of all the alder trees arching overhead. Where the road ends, go left onto the bark-mulch trail. And at the T junction, go left again on a path that brings you back to the viewpoint once more. Go downhill and straight ahead on the gravel path. At the next junction, go right along the northern side of the big pond.

The birds in and around the pond are easy to notice. Among them are ducks, coots and red-winged blackbirds. But it's easy to overlook a very important plant inhabitant of the pond that all these birds depend on: the cattail.

When you've finished checking out the cattails, birds and rabbits at Jericho Park, follow the path that goes back to the parking lot.

Cattails (Typha latifolia)

Cattails are the tall plants that grow around the edges and in the middle of the pond. Sometimes they can grow taller than people. The leaves are long and flat. The flowers of the cattail don't look like most flowers you see—they are crammed into the velvety brown spike at the top of the stem.

Many birds, such as red-winged blackbirds and marsh wrens, make their nests among cattails. In addition, some mammals, such as muskrats, live among the cattails, and some animals, including muskrats and geese, also eat parts of the cattail. Many years ago, First Nations peoples used cattails for all kinds of things: they ate the roots, young leaves and young flowers; they wove the leaves and steams into mats, blankets and clothing; and they even used the fluff from when the flowers go to seed as stuffing for pillows and for diapers.

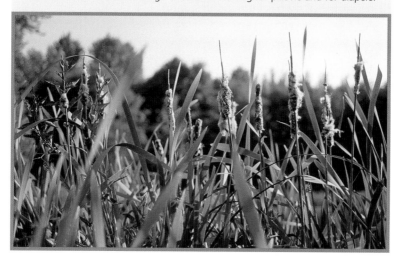

Pacific Spirit Park South

Length: 5.5-km loop

Time needed: 2.5 to 3 hours

Season: Year-round

Rating: Easy

Dogs: Yes, on leash

Stroller-friendly: All-terrain strollers only

Washrooms: At park centre, next to parking lot

Highlights: Salal, sword fern, Cutthroat Creek

Access: Follow 16th Avenue westward toward University of BC. About 1 kilometre past Blanca Street, look for Pacific Spirit Regional Park Centre on your right. Park in lot.

Driving time: 20 minutes

Pacific Spirit Regional Park has more than 50 kilometres of trails, which means lots of paths for lots of different hikes. This particular hike takes a route that shows just some of the different kinds of habitat within the park's 750 hectares of forest.

Your first stop should be the park centre facility, where you can pick up a map that shows all the trails in the park. With map in hand, head east for about 200 metres on a paved path that runs parallel to 16th Avenue. Then, beneath the power poles, look for the sign for the Salal Trail. Go through the gap in the wooden fence to start on this hikers-only path. Ferns, huckleberry bushes and vine maples line the trail. True to the trail's name, salal is everywhere on the forest floor here. You can eat salal berries, but not everyone likes their taste.

A few minutes later on the Salal Trail, you will reach a trail intersection. Go left onto the Lily of the Valley Trail. As you walk along, you can't help noticing all the big, burned-out stumps.

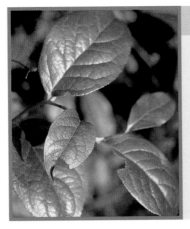

Salal (Gaultheria shallon)

Salal is one of the most common shrubs in coastal BC forests. It is an evergreen, which means that its leaves are green all year.

In spring and early summer, tiny, white flowers dangle from salal shrubs; in autumn they become purple berries. First Nations people ate salal berries fresh and dried and even dipped in fish grease. These days you might see salal leaves used in florist bouquets.

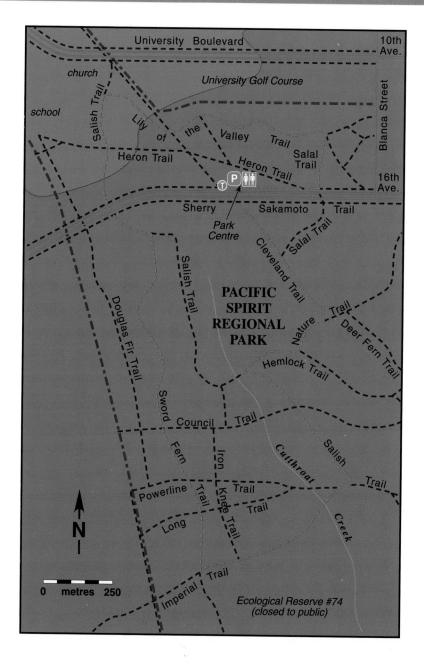

You will soon come to the intersection with the Cleveland Trail. Continue straight on the Lily of the Valley Trail for another 10 minutes to the Salish Trail. Turn left. Watch for mountain bikers and the occasional horseback rider on this multi-use trail.

Cutthroat Creek

This creek is a tributary of Musqueam Creek, which is another creek in the park. They are two of a very few old streams in Vancouver that were never filled in or re-routed. Still, the creeks have been damaged by the effects of such things as logging, sewage runoff and contamination by dog and horse poop.

In recent years, however, the Musqueam Band, community volunteers and the David Suzuki Foundation (with money from the federal and provincial governments and BC Hydro) have helped to restore the creek. Volunteers removed more than 400 kilograms of trash. They also planted more than 6000 trees along the creek to provide shade and reduce the creek's summer temperature to be more salmon- and trout-friendly.

In 1998, 28 coho salmon returned to the creek to spawn, which is a big improvement over 1996, when only six coho returned.

Follow the Salish Trail to 16th Avenue, cross the road and look for the continuation of the Salish Trail on the other side (just to the left). About 200 metres from the road, you will reach the junction with the Sword Fern Trail. Go right.

Sword Fern Trail is a hikers-only trail. You'll soon come to a boardwalk that takes you over some marshy areas. Notice that a lot of ferns grow on the forest floor. One type is the sword fern, the most common fern in the coastal rainforest (see p. 31).

Keep walking south on the Sword Fern Trail. You'll pass the Council Trail, the Powerline Trail and the Long Trail. When you come to the multi-use Imperial Trail, go left. (Watch for mountain bikes and horses.)

As you walk along this wide-open path, you may notice the occasional sign that tells you that the forest on the right is part of Ecological Reserve No. 74. This part of the park was set aside to provide a second-growth forest ecosystem close to the University of BC for study purposes. Only people involved in research or education projects may enter the reserve.

Salal Trail

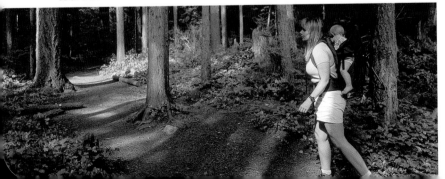

After walking for about 15 minutes, you'll reach tiny Cutthroat Creek, which was named for an endangered species of cutthroat trout that is about the size of an adult's finger. Don't walk in the creek or let your dogs run in it, because you could damage the trout's habitat.

Continue along the Imperial Trail to where it becomes a wider road. A little farther along there is a sign for the Salish Trail. Go left here and continue past the Council Trail until you come to the Hemlock Trail. Now go right. Several different kinds of trees surround you—Douglas-fir, western redcedar, Sitka spruce—in addition to the western hemlock that gives this trail its name.

Where the Hemlock Trail meets the Nature Trail, go left. A little bit farther along, where the Nature Trail meets the Cleveland Trail, go left again. Soon, you'll arrive back at 16th Avenue, right across the road from the park centre.

Sword Fern *(Polystichum munitum)*

Sword fern grows in clumps and has long fronds that, not surprisingly, look like swords. Ferns, unlike trees, shrubs and many other plants, use spores instead of seeds to reproduce. Look on the underside of the fronds for the spores—they look like round, brownish dots.

The sword fern was an important plant for the First Nations peoples of BC. Its fronds were used as a kind of lining in food storage boxes, in baskets and on berry-drying racks. But the sword fern's rhizome—a kind of underground stem—was even more important than the leaves. In times of famine, native peoples would dig up the rhizome, roast or steam it, then peel it and eat it. The top of the rhizome can be seen coming out of the soil. Look for the reddish-brown, scaly, woody clump at the base of the fronds.

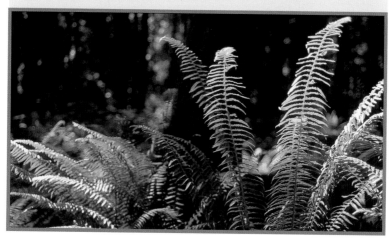

Towers Beach

Length: 4 km

Time needed: 2 to 2.5 hours

Season: October to April

Note: During the warmer months the area is a popular place for nude sunbathing.

Rating: Easy

Dogs: Yes, on leash

Stroller-friendly: No

Washrooms: Outhouses at trailhead, below parking lot

Highlights: Seaweed, diving ducks and mussels, harbour seals, searchlight towers

Access: Follow Northwest Marine Drive past Locarno and Spanish Banks beaches to the parking lot at Acadia Beach (where the road begins heading uphill toward the University of BC).

Driving time: 20 minutes

Vancouver is a seaside city, but the shoreline walks that most people do are on pavement—the seawalls—and not on the beach itself. Just beyond the city's westernmost edge, though, there are kilometres and kilometres of beach without seawalls. This hike takes in some of the best that Point Grey's beaches have to offer, from marine life to local history.

Seaweed

More than 600 different kinds of seaweed (large algae) live and grow in BC waters. They come in different shapes, sizes and colours—from green to red to yellow to purple. Many ocean animals, including snails, crabs, shrimp, fish, ducks and sea stars, depend on seaweed for food and shelter.

One of the most common kinds of seaweed is rockweed. As the name suggests, rockweed often attaches itself to rocks, and it frequently grows where it is above the water level much of the day.

Rockweed is also known by other names, such as 'bladder wrack' and 'popping wrack.' The first parts of these two names refer to the bulbous ends of the seaweed, which are filled with air and act like floats or bladders and which make a popping sound when crushed. These bulbous ends also produce the spores that rockweed uses to reproduce.

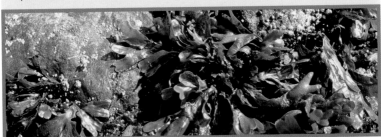

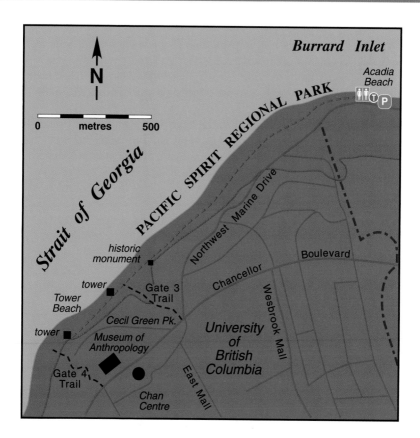

From the parking area, follow the trail down toward the waters of English Bay and head left along the beach. Across the water, you can see tiny Passage Island almost straight ahead. Bowen Island is the big landmass to the left, and just behind it are some of the mountains of the Sunshine Coast.

The trail passes by maple and alder trees across a small, often slippery bridge. Where the trail forks, go right. From here, your hiking will be on the beach. Where it's sandy, the walking is easy. But, where there are rocks, be careful because they can be slimy, or, in winter, frosty.

When you come to a rocky part of the beach, stop and look more closely at the different kinds of seaweed (see p. 32).

Walk a bit farther and find a comfortable log for a break. As you look out over the water, use binoculars to get a closer look at all those black dots bobbing on the waves. You'll notice that most of them are ducks—sea ducks that overwinter on the coast and get their food under the waves (see p. 35).

You may also have noticed that some of those black dots you are seeing on the water aren't ducks. Some are floating logs, and others look like dogs out for a swim. But they're not dogs, they're harbour seals (see p. 34).

Since you've already had a good look at the beach beneath your feet and what's going on in the water, turn your attention to the cliffs and trees as you continue your hike. You might see a bald eagle perched high on a western redcedar tree. And you'll probably also notice some mudslides and uprooted trees.

The Iona Jetty, a short distance to the south, has changed the direction of the cliffside water currents. As a result, the cliffs are being eroded bit by bit every year. More and more of the mud, sand and clay that was deposited here by the Fraser River over thousands of years is being carried away.

As you come around a bit of a corner, you will see the first of the two towers that give Towers Beach its name (see p. 35).

If you continue past a big berm of smooth, rounded river stones brought here to help control cliff erosion, you'll see the second tower. And you'll also get good views across Georgia Strait to the Gulf Islands and Vancouver Island. Then, when you're ready, retrace your steps to Acadia Beach.

Harbour Seal *(Phoca vitulina)*

During December, January and February, there are large numbers of harbour seals just off the beach. Marine biologists are uncertain about why the seals like to gather in this area. But they have noticed that in winter the seals spend more time in the water than they do on shore.

The seals have been seen in the waters off Point Grey for a very long time. The native peoples who lived in the Vancouver area long before the first European settlers had a legend about one particular seal that was the biggest anyone had ever seen.

In *Legends of Vancouver*, Pauline Johnson tells how a chief decided to hunt this 'king of seals.' From his canoe, the chief threw a spear (attached to a long cedar rope) and hit the giant seal. But the seal was so big and so powerful that, as it plunged into the sea and tried to get away, it ended up dragging the chief and his canoe behind. In the end, the seal jumped high into the air and dove deep into the water with such force that it ripped the rope

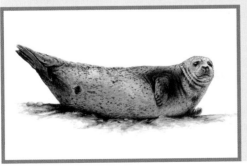

right out of the chief's hands and disappeared.

A year later, the chief found the seal's body at Deer Lake but was never able to find the river that the seal used to access the lake. How the seal got to Deer Lake remains unknown.

Sea Ducks

Some of the sea duck species that you might see here are the surf scoter, harlequin duck, common and Barrow's goldeneyes, bufflehead and old-squaw. Some, such as the surf scoter and the goldeneyes, often hang out together in huge flocks. Others, such as the harlequin duck, tend to gather in smaller groups.

Sea ducks can dive as deep as the sea bottom in search of food: fish, shell-fish (mussels), crustaceans (crabs, shrimp) and seaweed. When a sea duck eats a mussel, it swallows the mussel shell and all. Once swallowed, the shell is 'chewed' to pieces by the duck's gizzard, a muscular part of the stomach that is lined with ridges or hard plates. Think of a gizzard as a bird's teeth, only they are in the stomach, not in the mouth. Other birds use their gizzards to grind up other hard foodstuffs, such as nuts and hard-shelled grains.

Searchlight Towers

When Canada was involved in the Second World War (1939–45), the government was concerned that Vancouver could be the target of enemy attacks. In response, they built the 'Point Grey Battery': a collection of searchlight towers, big guns and underground storage places filled with ammunition.

No enemy attacks ever took place, but a freighter anchored in Burrard Inlet was once hit by a warning shot that had ricocheted off a fishing boat that cruised into the inlet unaware of the wartime crisis.

Searchlight tower

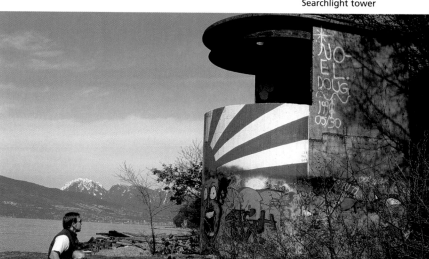

Capilano Canyon

Length: 4.5-km loop

Time needed: 2 to 2.5 hours

Season: Year-round

Rating: Moderate; elevation gain of 50 metres

Dogs: Yes, on leash

Stroller-friendly: No

Washrooms: At parking lot near dam; at hatchery

Highlights: Dam, giant trees, canyon, hatchery

Access: Take the Lions Gate Bridge to North Vancouver. Take the eastbound ramp to Marine Drive, turn left onto Capilano Road and follow it all the way up to the Cleveland Dam parking lot for Capilano River Regional Park.

Driving time: 25 minutes

Capilano Canyon has been one of my favourite destinations since I was a kid. The trails pass big trees and steep canyon walls, and they cross bridges over crystal-clear pools and treacherous rapids. This scenic figure-eight loop takes in the best that Capilano Canyon has to offer.

From the parking area, go west to the Cleveland Dam. On the right is Capilano Lake; in the distance at the lake's end are the twin peaks of the Lions.

Cross the dam. A gravel clearing is at the far end. Go left to take the trail that dips downward. At the next fork, about 50 metres farther on, go left again, continuing downhill.

You will soon come to a trail junction. Stay left (the Capilano Pacific Trail goes right) and head downhill for another 25 metres to the Giant Fir Trail. Take the stairs on the left. At the bottom of the stairs stands a huge Douglas-fir tree known as 'Grandfather Capilano' (see p. 39).

The Cleveland Dam

If you came to Capilano Canyon before 1954, there would have been no lake. Back then, before the dam was built, a suspension bridge crossed the steep canyon at this location. It was decided that the growing population of the Lower Mainland needed a new water supply, however, so the Capilano River was dammed.

Cleveland Dam, named after Ernest Cleveland, the first commissioner of the Greater Vancouver Water District, was completed in 1954. It took a year for Capilano Lake to fill to its current size of 5 kilometres long and almost 1 kilometre wide.

Under all that water lie trees, parts of a hotel, a house, a cable-car, a log flume and perhaps a memento or two left behind by early mountaineers who traversed the valley on their way to the Lions.

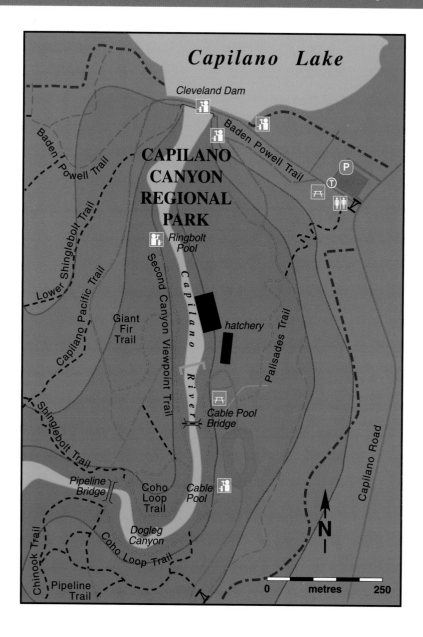

Before you continue, also notice the size of the fallen tree next to Grandfather, as well as the old snag behind that's riddled with woodpecker holes. Follow the trail until you reach a T junction. Go left and wander through a lush rainforest understorey of huckleberry, salal and salmonberry. You will approach more wooden fencing and two more big trees.

When the trail reaches the riverside, go left to the Second Canyon Viewpoint for a different perspective of Cleveland Dam. After a look, turn around and retrace your steps to the last junction, but continue straight instead of going back uphill.

At the next junction, continue straight ahead along the river. You will come to a wooden bridge from which you can often see people fishing in the river. Go left over the bridge. Sometimes you might see daring whitewater kayakers playing in the water below.

At the next T junction, go right over a small footbridge and past a marshy area with skunk cabbage and old stumps to follow the Coho

Cleveland Dam

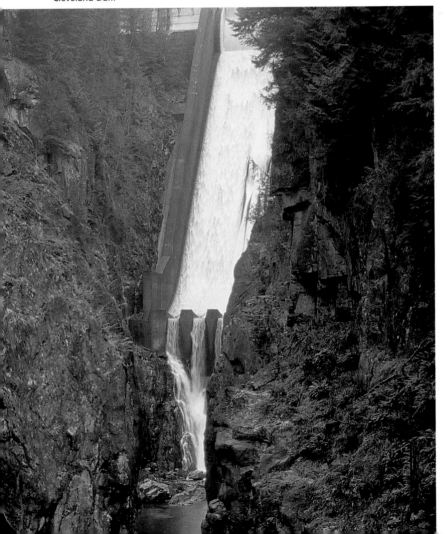

Grandfather Capilano

This tree stands 61 metres tall—taller than 30 tall men standing one on top of the other—and 7.5 metres around. Although this tree is big, there were once many more trees of this size and bigger here. Most of these forest giants were cut down in the late 1800s. One report tells of a western redcedar that when cut down measured more than 19 metres around.

Grandfather Capilano is about 600 years old. This tree has managed to survive logging and fires and probably the invasion of an insect or two, but a fence had to be built around it to save it from getting trampled upon by people. The weight of all the people who used to walk close to this giant tree was starting to crush its roots. That's why you should stay behind the fence.

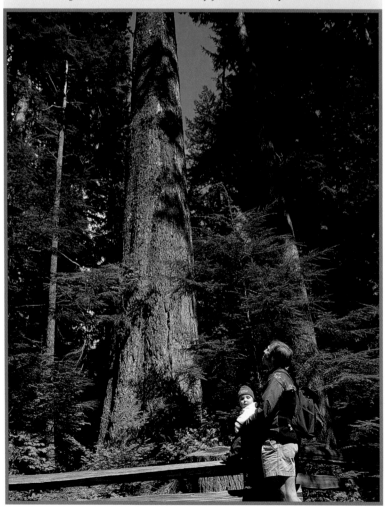

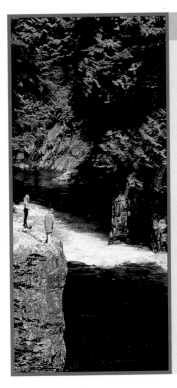

The Canyon Walls

About 15,000 years ago, the Capilano Canyon didn't exist. In fact, neither did the Capilano River. Both came into being only at the end of the last ice age, or 'glaciation.'

Way back then, a huge glacier had scraped out a broad valley north of the present Capilano Canyon. When the glacier started to melt, gravel piled up where the edge of the glacier had been, and water collected into a lake behind the rocks. In time the water spilled over, but at a point that was actually east of the present Capilano River.

Where the dam is now, a solid rock barrier existed. Over time, however, the water wore away the rock until it found a fault in it. In a process that took many years, the water began to flow out of the lake through the eroded rock. As the water pounded away, it carved the steep canyon walls that you see today.

Loop Trail. A bit farther along there is some wooden fencing on the right and the Cable Pool Trail. You can take this trail right down to the river for a look, or you can wander just as far as the wooden platform and benches—a good place for a snack or a break.

Return to the main trail and go right to continue along the Coho Loop Trail. At first the trail climbs uphill. Then you go down a set of stairs. Go straight ahead, ignoring any side trails. You then go up another set of stairs and gradually climb uphill past more trees, a lush understorey and river viewpoints. The trail soon tops out and heads back downhill. You will go down some more stairs and cross two bridges before you come to a trail junction. Go right to reach the Pipeline Bridge, below which is Dog Leg Canyon.

Cross the bridge and go right, then right again to continue along the Coho Loop Trail as it hugs the clifftops overlooking the canyon. This beautiful little part of the forest seems always to have birds twittering and singing. Continue on the clifftop-hugging trail and you will arrive back at the Cable Pool's wooden bridge. Cross it, but this time go left toward the parking area and the Capilano River Hatchery.

When you're finished looking around the hatchery, go left and head toward the 'mushroom bench'—an old stump with a bench and a roof built onto it. A bit to the left of the 'mushroom' is the trail back to the top of the Cleveland Dam.

Almost all of this final kilometre is uphill. The first section is a steady climb through a beautiful forest to a gravel road. Go left, staying along the lower fork of the road. At the next fork, go right to take the upper gravel road. At the top of the hill, it's worth going left for a short side trip to a viewpoint right alongside the dam.

After taking in the magnificent view, retrace your steps to the fork, go left toward the dam and climb the final flight of stairs. The parking area lies straight ahead.

The Capilano River Hatchery

The hatchery, built in 1971, is here to help make up for the changes that we humans have made to the river and the salmon that live in it. Before the dam was built, coho salmon and steelhead trout swam upstream to reproduce at the places where they had hatched. After the dam was built, though, the fish had no way to return to their original spawning grounds.

These days, coho and chinook salmon and steelhead trout are raised at the hatchery and released downstream of the dam so that they can swim to the ocean. Although most of the working parts of the hatchery (the incubation boxes and rearing ponds, for example) are closed to the public, there are displays at the hatchery that show you what goes on behind the scenes. Depending on when you come, you can see either young salmon getting ready to head out or adult salmon jumping up the fish ladder on their way to try to spawn.

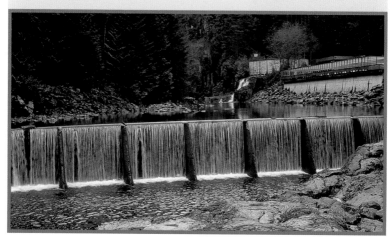

Lynn Canyon

Length: 3-km loop

Time needed: 1 to 2 hours

Season: Year-round

Rating: Moderate; some steep sections

Dogs: Yes, on leash

Stroller-friendly: No

Washrooms: At park entrance, near the suspension bridge

Highlights: Moss, water erosion, suspension bridge, ecology centre

Access: From Highway 1 (Upper Levels Highway), take the Lynn Valley Road exit and head north to Peters Road, where you turn right. Follow the signs to Lynn Canyon Park and park in the lot.

Driving time: 35 minutes

The hiking at Lynn Canyon is good in just about any season and any weather. On hot summer days, the forest and river keep the trails cool; on wet winter days, everything looks so lush and green that you can almost forget about the grey skies.

From the parking area, follow the paved road as it loops southward. Look for a yellow gate that marks the start of an old service road. Go left and follow the wide gravel path as it slopes gently downward. If you look at the trunks of the trees on both sides of the path, you will notice moss growing on them.

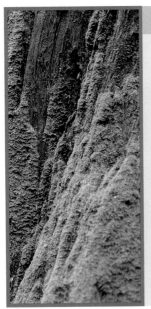

Moss on Trees

Moss grows on trees for a couple of reasons.

First, trees usually don't go anywhere. Moss needs a stable place to grow, which is why it also grows on rocks, stumps and basically anything that stays around long enough for a moss spore to settle and grow.

Secondly, moss likes moisture, of which there is usually plenty in a rainforest. That's also why, in open forests of this kind, the moss often grows on the north side of a tree. Because BC lies north of the equator, the north side of a tree generally gets less sun than the south side. With less sun, it is more likely to remain damp, which is good for moss. In denser forests, where sunlight can't penetrate the tree cover as easily, you'll see moss growing on all sides of a tree trunk.

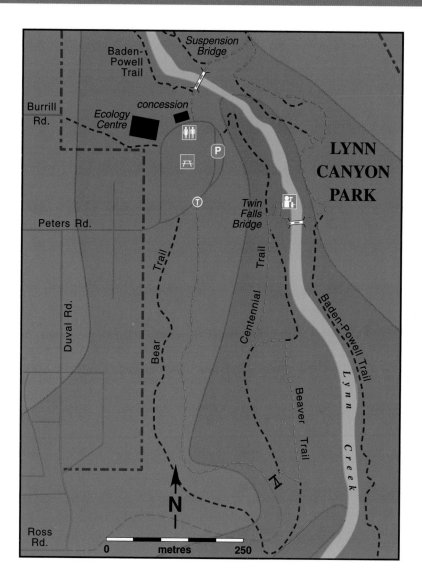

Continue along the gravel path. About 100 metres from the start, a trail branches to the right. Follow it past another gate and then make a left turn onto Beaver Trail, which drops down into lush forest.

Cross two small bridges over small feeder streams that trickle into Lynn Creek. When you reach a junction, go straight (north) along the main trail. (The trail that goes right leads down to the creek.) A short, steep uphill section will bring you back to Centennial Trail.

When you reach a clearing, look on the right for a long set of stairs. Follow them down toward Twin Falls Bridge. Just before the bridge is a

Water Erosion

Unlike the Capilano and Seymour rivers, Lynn Creek isn't controlled by a dam. As a result, the creek can sometimes run really high—in spring, for example, when mountain snow is melting, or after a long, hard rain. At other times, such as at the end of a long, dry summer, it can be just a trickle.

Regardless of its level, there's always water in Lynn Creek and it's always working away at the rocks in the creekbed. The water gets a helping hand from tiny stones that get carried along. These stones scour the rocky surfaces of the creekbed like sandpaper on a piece of wood.

A pothole forms when a round stone happens to roll into a little depression in the rock where there is an eddy or whirlpool in the creek. The water current makes the stone go around and around, making the depression bigger and bigger over time.

Lynn Creek

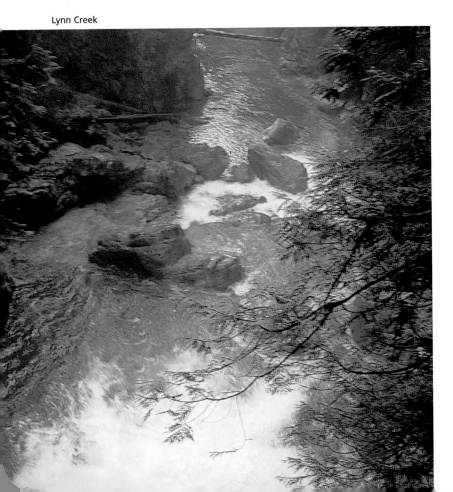

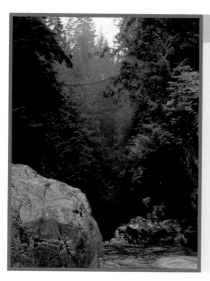

The Suspension Bridge

At one time, the only way to cross Lynn Creek was on logs—without handrails. In 1912, a suspension bridge was built, and back then you had to pay 10¢ to cross. The bridge wasn't maintained, however, and eventually it had to be closed.

Later, the District of North Vancouver took over the bridge, repaired it and re-opened it. Today this bridge, which stands 50 metres above Lynn Creek (about the same height as a 12-storey building), is free for the crossing.

viewpoint where you can see great big boulders worn smooth by water as well as places where potholes have been carved into the rock (see p. 44).

Continue to Twin Falls Bridge. Before this bridge was built in 1930, the only way to cross the river was on a big tree that was felled across the creek. Below is a big pool of water. Sometimes people jump into the pool to swim, but it is very dangerous to do so, because the river's current is strong and unpredictable, and rocks lie near the surface in places. Many people have died here.

Once you've reached the other side of the bridge, go up the wooden stairs. Follow the signs, more trail and more stairs until finally you reach the Lynn Canyon Suspension Bridge.

Once you have crossed the suspension bridge, you're back in the parking area where you started. But, before heading home, go right and make a visit to the Lynn Canyon Ecology Centre.

The Lynn Canyon Ecology Centre

At the Lynn Valley Ecology Centre you can explore nature indoors! There are lots of things to see and touch that help you to learn more about the rainforest and the plants and animals that live there. The ecology centre also has puppet shows and nature films and offers programs where naturalists show you different parts of the park.

For information on programs or on the centre's hours, call (604) 981-3103.

Lynn Headwaters

Length: 6-km loop

Time needed: 2.5 to 3 hours

Season: Year-round

Rating: Moderate; elevation gain of 225 metres

Dogs: Yes, on leash

Stroller-friendly: No

Washrooms: Outhouses at park entrance

Highlights: Big stumps, views, glacial erratics, deciduous trees

Access: From Highway 1 (Upper Levels Highway), take the Lynn Valley Road exit and head north. Stay on Lynn Valley Road, past the turn-off for Lynn Canyon Park, until you get to its very end. Then follow the green and yellow signs to the parking lots.

Driving time: 30 minutes

The trails of Lynn Headwaters Regional Park lead you to all sorts of beautiful terrain, including fragrant groves of alder and aspen, cedar-spired forest cathedrals, skunky-scented marsh and, of course, the clear, rushing waters of Lynn Creek.

From the parking area, cross the bridge over Lynn Creek and go right on the gravel road. After a few minutes of walking, look on the left for the beginning of the Lynn Loop Trail just before the yellow gate that marks the boundary between Lynn Headwaters and the Lower Seymour Conservation Reserve.

Follow the trail uphill for a bit. It soon levels off and wanders through a mossy forest filled with both living trees and old stumps and snags.

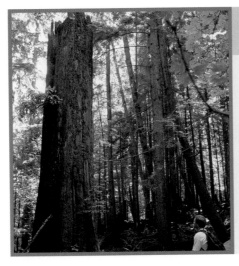

Big Stumps & Big Trees

The stumps are all that remain of trees logged here in the early 1900s. Some of these trees were so big that they grew as tall as some of the office buildings today in downtown Vancouver. One Douglas-fir tree was said to be 120 metres high, making it taller than the Marine Building at the corner of Burrard and Hastings.

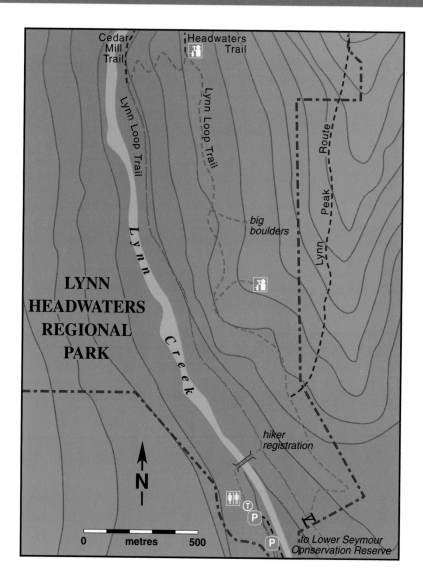

After checking out the stumps, continue straight ahead. (Another trail branches right to Lynn Peak.) In a few minutes you will pass the remains of an old cabin, now covered with ferns, moss and other forest plants. A 15-minute hike farther along the trail will take you to a huge snag (the standing remains of a big tree). Next to it there is a side trail that leads to a viewpoint. Follow it up, up, up, and in about 15 minutes you will come to a rocky bluff (see p. 48).

After you've had a water break and a good look around the bluff, retrace your steps down to the main trail and continue northward.

About 20 minutes later, after passing several tiny creeks and crossing bridge No. 17, you come to another side trail. Go right and follow the trail to two huge boulders, both about 7 metres high, that were brought here by glaciers between 12,000 and 25,000 years ago.

Return to the main trail and keep walking through the green beauty of the forest. About five minutes of walking brings you to a big upended stump. As you imagine what it would be like to walk through a forest of such big trees, don't forget to look for a trail on the left. Follow this trail down stairs and switchbacks for about 10 minutes to get back down to Lynn Creek. Then go left.

The species of trees in the forest here are different from the forest that you walked through earlier. Up higher, the trees were mostly Douglas-fir, western redcedar and western hemlock—all coniferous trees. Here, the trees are mostly alder, aspen and bigleaf maple—all deciduous trees.

After walking along the creekside trail for about 20 minutes, look on the right for the remains of an old truck with some alder trees growing right in the middle of it. It's left over from the area's logging days.

The View from the Bluff

Weather permitting, you can get a good view of the mountains and the city from the bluff. To your left, in the distance, is Coquitlam's Heritage Mountain. To the right of that are Burnaby Mountain and the Ironworkers Memorial Second Narrows Bridge. The lower Seymour Valley is below you. On a clear day, in the very far distance, you can even see the United States, with Mount Baker rising to the southeast and the San Juan Islands lying to the southwest.

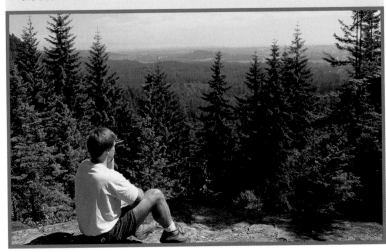

Glacial Erratics

Back when the global climate was very cold, glaciers extended from places farther north down through the Yukon and BC. At one time, the ice sheet here measured up to 1800 metres thick—higher than most of the mountains on the North Shore. As the glaciers moved, they pushed piles of rocks and dirt in front of them. Many of the rocks were crushed as they moved along, but some remained large. When the climate warmed up and the ice sheets melted, those big rocks were left behind.

So why are these boulders called 'erratics'? Well, 'erratic' means 'not regular,' and these boulders are not regular in that they are usually made of a different kind of rock than the normal bedrock of the area where they now reside.

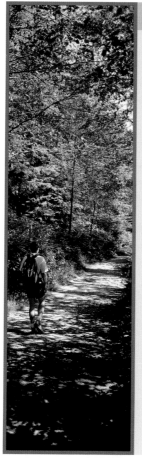

Coniferous & Deciduous Trees

What do people mean when they talk about coniferous trees and deciduous trees? One of the best clues can be found in the words themselves.

The word 'coniferous' means 'cone-bearing,' so coniferous trees have cones. Some trees, such as the western hemlock, have tiny cones only as big as a medium-sized grape. Others, such as the ponderosa pine of the BC Interior, can have cones as big as large apples. There are other ways to identify conifers, as they are also called. For instance, they typically have needles instead of flat leaves, and almost all coniferous trees keep their needles year-round, so they are also often called 'evergreens.'

The word 'deciduous' comes from a Latin word meaning 'to fall,' so, as you would expect, deciduous trees have leaves that fall off every autumn. So if you see a tree that doesn't have any leaves in winter, it's a deciduous tree. Most trees that have leaves instead of needles are deciduous.

Larch trees are the only exception to the rule. Larches are conifers with cones and needles, but in autumn their needles turn yellow and fall off, so they are also deciduous. (Larch trees don't grow wild near the coast, but both the western larch and the alpine larch grow in the BC Interior.)

Maplewood Flats

Length: 2.5-km loop

Time needed: 1 to 2 hours

Season: Year-round

Rating: Easy

Dogs: No

Stroller-friendly: Yes

Washrooms: Near entrance in Pacific Environmental Science Centre building

Highlights: Bridge, osprey nests, dragonflies, freshwater ponds

Access: Take Highway 1 (Upper Levels Highway) to the north end of the Second Narrows Bridge and take the eastbound exit for Deep Cove. Follow Dollarton Highway for 2 kilometres and watch for the wildlife viewing signs. The entrance to Maplewood Flats is on the right, just across from the Crab Shack. A few parking spots are available within the compound; otherwise, you'll have to use the parking area on Dollarton and walk in.

Driving time: 25 minutes

One of the best-kept secrets on the North Shore, Maplewood Flats is a sanctuary for both birds and bird-lovers. More than 200 bird species have been spotted, from tiny rufous hummingbirds to large trumpeter swans. The habitat also attracts a variety of other wildlife, including dragonflies, butterflies, frogs, otters and deer.

Start your walk with a visit to the sanctuary office. The sanctuary warden can tell you what kinds of animal species you might spot and about some of the activities that happen at Maplewood Flats.

Next head past the fenced area where a small garden of native plants grows. These plants, which help attract birds and butterflies, get replanted all around the flats.

The path continues past blackberry bushes that attract small songbirds. The birds love blackberries and hide among the brambles and leaves. In just a few minutes, you will arrive at a bridge (see p. 53); take some time here to see what wildlife is around.

Finish crossing the bridge and take the path on the left. In summer the path is lined with buttercups, clover, lupines, lots of shrubs and little trees. Songbirds love this area, and you can see them flitting back and forth in search of food and sometimes nesting materials.

At the next junction, go left, then left again down a side trail to a beach covered in driftwood. Look out over the water—or mud-flats, if it's low tide—to find a row of five pilings. On top of the last piling is a nest made by osprey (see p. 52). If you look through binoculars, you'll see what looks like a big pile of sticks.

In April, May or even June look for a pair of osprey on or near the nest at the end of the pilings. You might also see the heads of some osprey chicks. If

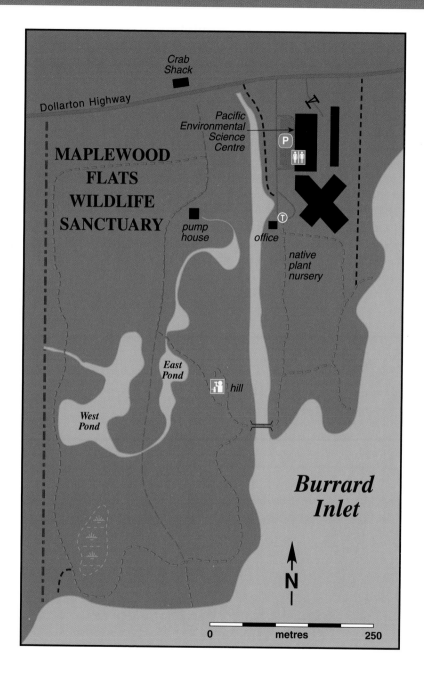

you're really lucky, you could see an osprey catch a fish. This beautiful bird hovers above the water until it spots a fish swimming below, then it swoops down and plucks the fish right out of the water with its sharp talons.

Return to the last junction and go left. In summer the path is lined with bright red bursts of crimson clover. In late summer, be sure to check the leaves of the blackberry bushes on the left of the trail for tiny Pacific treefrogs. A bit farther on, the ground gets marshy. Here you can see cattails and hear and see red-winged blackbirds. From spring through autumn you can also see other creatures that love the marsh—dragonflies (see p. 54).

At the next junction, a side trail goes left to a remnant of salt-marsh. At one time the entire shoreline from Deep Cove to Ambleside was salt-marsh. Now, because of industrial and residential growth, this tiny fragment is all that is left. It may not look like much, but it's very important—it provides food and shelter to many different plants and animals.

Return to the main trail and follow the path to the freshwater ponds (see p. 55). Then continue along the path and into the woods. Alder and cottonwood trees mix with salmonberry shrubs and wildflowers, such as herb-Robert.

Osprey *(Pandion haliaetus)*

The year 1989 marked the first time since the early 1900s that osprey had nested in this area.

One of the reasons that osprey disappeared here and in many other areas was a pesticide called DDT. Farmers used to use DDT to kill insects that were eating their crops, but DDT didn't stay only on the crops—it got into ponds, lakes, rivers and creeks and even poisoned parts of the sea. When birds ate insects or fish or any other food that had DDT in it, the chemical would

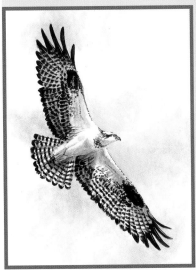

harm them, too. Even if there was not enough DDT in a female bird to kill it, the shells of her eggs were often so thin that they would break before the baby birds were old enough to hatch.

DDT was banned, and since then osprey and other birds have recovered. Osprey like Maplewood Flats because it has good nesting locations and because there are lots of fish in relatively shallow water.

In May of every second year the Wild Bird Trust celebrates with a Return of the Osprey Festival where you can learn about osprey and other birds seen at Maplewood Flats.

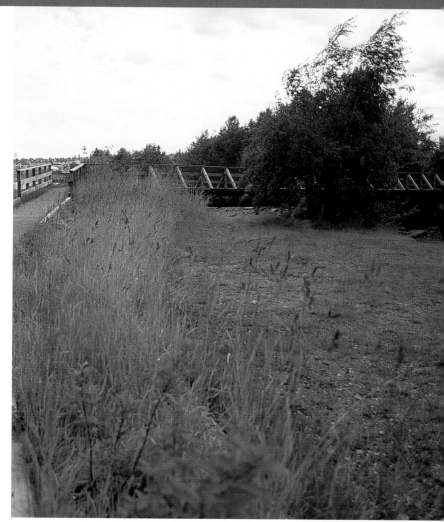

Bridge at Maplewood

The Bridge Viewpoint

Take a few minutes to stand in the middle of the bridge and observe your surroundings. If you look north, you might spot a river otter slinking up the muddy banks of the slough. Or you might see a kingfisher swoop down from a nearby branch and pluck a fish out of the water. If you lean over the bridge railing at high tide, you might see mergansers or other diving ducks swimming underwater in search of fish.

And, if you turn around and look out toward Burrard Inlet, you might see other kinds of marine life, including gulls, sea ducks and harbour seals.

At the junction, go right. A bit farther along, go right again onto an old dirt road. Then make one more right onto another old road. About 5 to 10 minutes later, watch on the left for a path. Take it, and follow it past another freshwater pond.

At the next junction, go left and up a small hill for a good overview of this part of Maplewood Flats and parts beyond. Then retrace your steps down the hill, go left at the junction and retrace your steps to the bridge.

Cross the bridge. If you want to do a little bit more walking, go right at the next pathway instead of straight back to the parking area. You'll see more of the mud-flats, more birds and more insects—and maybe even a harbour seal or two. After following the path for about 10 minutes, you'll be back at the sanctuary office.

Dragonflies (Order Odonata)

In some ways, dragonflies are even more prehistoric than dinosaurs. Scientists have found fossils of dragonflies (and their close relatives the damselflies) that are as much as 300 million years old.

Of the 5000 species of dragonflies in the world, about 80 can be found in BC. The smallest ones are no longer than a sewing needle, and the largest are about as long as a crayon. Dragonflies come in many colours, including red, blue, green, orange and yellow.

Dragonflies have four wings that each move independently. These bugs can fly forward and backward. They can fly up and down. What a dragonfly can't do with its wings is fold them against its body. These wings are very powerful, but they are also very fragile, so don't try to catch dragonflies. Just enjoy watching them.

All dragonflies are hunters. Lucky for us, one of their favourite foods is mosquitoes.

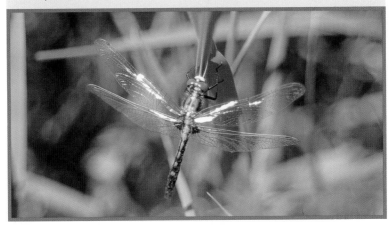

Freshwater Ponds

These ponds were created by people to replace some of the natural wetland habitat that has been lost to housing and industry. According to a 1996 publication by the West Coast Environmental Law Research Foundation, about 75 percent of the wetlands that once existed in the Lower Mainland have been lost to development.

Freshwater ponds attract different species of animals than salt-marshes do. For example, some ducks visit only freshwater ponds and lakes because that's where they find the kind of food that they eat. Other birds need specific freshwater wetland plants, such as cattails, for nesting.

Before the ponds were made here, this area was just a jumble of broken chunks of concrete, pipes and puddles. Now the area has a stable supply of fresh water, native plants grow here again, nesting boxes have been installed and there are all kinds of insect species that many birds love to eat.

Freshwater pond

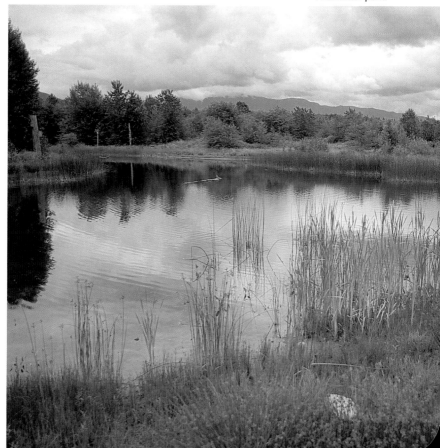

Lower Seymour Conservation Reserve

Length: 5-km loop

Time needed: 2 to 2.5 hours

Season: Year-round

Rating: Moderate; one steep uphill section at end with elevation gain of 100 metres

Dogs: No

Stroller-friendly: All-terrain strollers only

Washrooms: Outhouses, near the Learning Lodge

Highlights: Deer, Seymour River, tunnel, homesteads

Access: Follow Highway 1 (Upper Levels Highway) to just north of the Second Narrows Bridge and take the Lillooet Road exit. Follow Lillooet Road north past Capilano College and past the cemetery. Stay on this road, which is now gravel, until you get to the parking area.

Driving time: 45 minutes

Whether it's a cool, rainy day in December or a hot, sunny day in July, the Lower Seymour Conservation Reserve is a perfect destination. This hike follows trails through the forest and along the Seymour River. On the way are reminders of the people who once lived here.

Head to the northeast corner of the main parking area to find a gravel path that leads to a T junction. Then go right to follow the Twin Bridges Trail. On a quiet day you might be lucky enough to see deer here on the edges of the second-growth forest.

Very rarely, you might also see cougar here. That's because sometimes cougars eat deer. (They also eat rabbits, mice and birds.) While cougars are beautiful, they can also be dangerous (see p. 16).

Not much farther along you will arrive at the junction with the Homestead Trail. Go straight ahead, following the trail that goes to Twin Bridges. Notice the variety of plants. If you're here in spring or summer, you might see the tiny white foamflower and other wildflowers

Black-tailed Deer
(Odocoileus hemionus ssp. columbianus)

The species of deer that lives in this area is the black-tailed deer (a type of mule deer). The male can be as tall as, and weigh much more than, a typical adult human. The female is a little smaller than the male. The black-tailed deer ranges from reddish-brown to greyish-brown and has a black tip on its tail. It eats many kinds of plants, including the softer parts of trees (Douglas-fir, western redcedar) and shrubs (blackberry, huckleberry, salal).

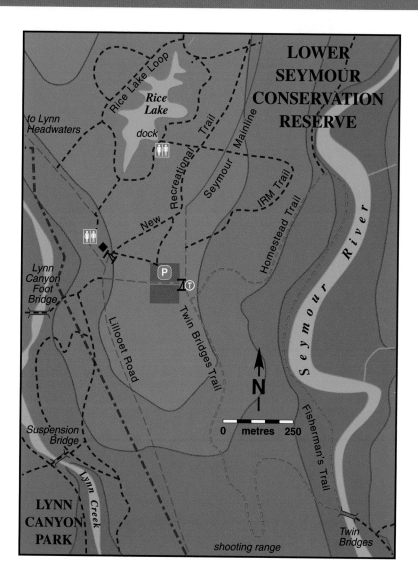

in bloom. The trees here are mostly smaller western hemlocks, but farther down the road there are bigger, taller Douglas-firs.

As the path continues its descent, you can hear rushing water. After a 30-minute or so hike from the junction, you will arrive at the Seymour River and Twin Bridges. Only one of the two bridges still stands. The foundations of the other bridge are just downstream.

From the junction, head north on the Fisherman's Trail. About 25 metres along on the right, a staircase will take you down to the river's edge for a short side trip.

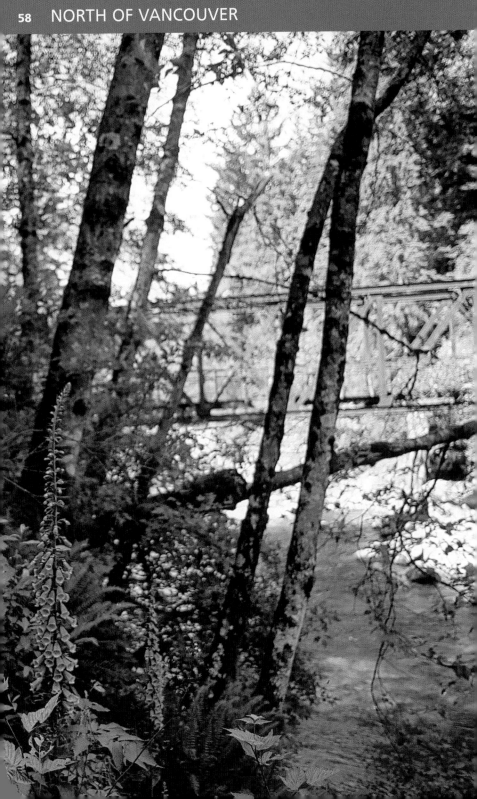

The Seymour River

The Seymour River starts high in the Coast Mountains. Melting snow feeds a lake called Loch Lomond, and its outflow is the start of the river.

Along the way, a number of tributary creeks—Clipper, Balfour and Sheba, to name a few—add their waters to the Seymour. They then pour into Seymour Lake, which was created when the Seymour Dam was built in 1928. (Seymour Lake, Capilano Lake and Coquitlam Lake together supply fresh water to much of the Lower Mainland.)

The amount of water in the lower part of the Seymour River can be controlled by opening or closing part of the dam. When the lake gets too high—because of rain or fast-melting snow in spring—more water can be let out. When people use more water during a long spell of hot weather, less water can be let out of the lake.

Return to the main trail and continue past salmonberry and red elderberry bushes for another 25 metres. You will come to a sign that explains what was happening here almost 100 years ago. On the other side of the trail, hidden in a rock bluff, is a tunnel (see p. 60).

As you continue, the foliage on the right opens to reveal views of the river. Then the trail enters a dense stand of red alder. Look on the right for evidence of some old cabins (see p. 61). In winter, when the shrubs and trees are leafless, it's easier to see the old fireplaces and gateposts. Right beside one old gatepost is an interpretive sign.

Continue along the trail until you reach a junction. The Fisherman's Trail continues straight ahead along the river for another 4.5 kilometres, but we'll go left onto the Homestead Trail. It's 1 kilometre to the top, with the trail rising gradually at first, then more steeply. The path soon levels, then rises gradually again. You will cross a small creek and then head steeply up again.

Soon, you're at the top again. Go right to find the gravel path leading back to the main parking area.

The Pipeline Tunnel

This tunnel is all that remains of the first water pipeline, built in 1908, to bring water from the Seymour River to the city of Vancouver. A dam was constructed, downstream from the one in use today. The section of pipeline that went from the dam to the start of the Seymour Canyon, a distance of about 6.5 kilometres, was made of Douglas-fir wood.

At what is now Twin Bridges (there was still only one bridge at that time) the wooden pipeline joined a steel pipeline that ran all the way down to Burrard Inlet. Although wood was cheaper to build with, steel was needed to withstand the increasing pressure as the water ran downhill. The water then fed through a pipe across the bottom of Burrard Inlet, where the Second Narrows Bridge now stands. The pipeline could transport 34 million litres of water each day.

By 1913, more water pressure was needed and so a second pipeline, entirely of steel, was built parallel to the first pipeline. Eventually the wood pipe rotted, but in winter, when the plants along the trail die back, it's still possible to see an occasional piece of metal that was used to bind the pipeline together.

Old tunnel

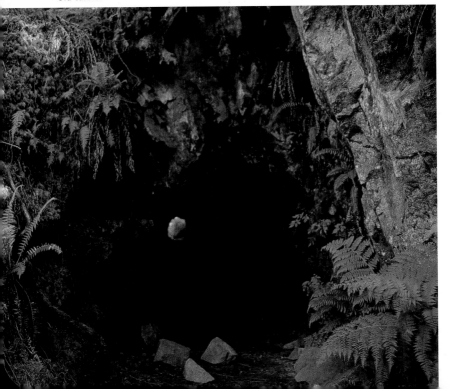

The Homesteads

A small settlement existed here in the 1920s and 1930s. There were already six houses when the Fowler family built an additional six cabins and rented them to tourists and fishermen. Residents and visitors could get supplies at either of two stores in the area. One was located south of Twin Bridges. The other, which stood just north of the bridges, featured a place where people could have afternoon tea while enjoying a view of the river.

The gatepost here stood in front of the Fowler family home, which boasted a vegetable garden and dairy cows. The family also owned property on the other side of the river and wanted to build more cabins. But in the 1950s the area was closed to protect the water supply from contamination.

Old homestead

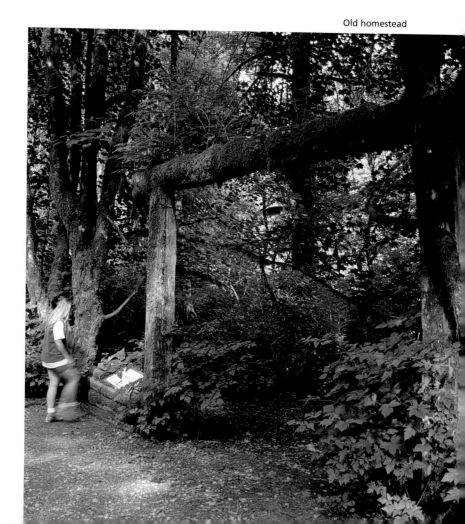

Dog Mountain

Length: 6 km

Time needed: 2.5 to 3 hours

Season: June to October

Rating: Moderate; rolling terrain with roots and rocks

Dogs: Yes, on leash

Stroller-friendly: No

Washrooms: At parking lot near beginning of hike

Highlights: Amabilis fir, chipmunks, grey jays, cabin remains

Access: Follow Highway 1 (Upper Levels Highway) to just north of the Second Narrows Bridge and take the exit for Mount Seymour and Lillooet Road. Keep right to get onto Mount Seymour Parkway and head eastward. At Parkgate Centre, turn left onto Mount Seymour Road and follow it to the large parking area at the very top.

Driving time: 45 minutes

Look for the BC Parks sign at the far corner of the parking lot. Then look for a wide gravel path that goes toward the trees. When you come to a post with a map, go left.

Now you're in the forest. Notice how many different species of trees there are. Each species has its own type of bark, needles and cone. In this forest there are three species of big tree: western hemlock, yellow-cedar and amabilis fir.

Amabilis Fir *(Abies amabilis)*

The easiest way to recognize an amabilis fir tree is by its needles. Amabilis fir needles are flat, with a little notch at the tip. The top part is a dark, shiny green. Turn the needle over and you should see two thin, silvery lines. In southwestern BC, amabilis fir trees grow only high in the mountains.

People have used this fir for many purposes. Native peoples used to chew the pitch (sticky sap) like chewing-gum. Explorers made tea from the needles, which are rich in vitamin C, to stay healthy on long voyages. These days amabilis fir is used mainly as lumber to build houses and furniture.

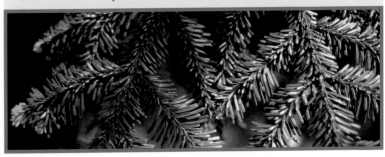

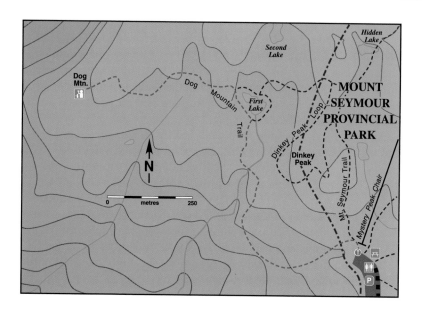

Yellow-pine Chipmunk *(Tamias amoenus)*

These little guys eat seeds and fruit. If you share a snack (no baked goods or candy, please) with a chipmunk, you can see how it stuffs food into pouches in its cheeks. These pouches allow it to carry food back to a quiet, safe place where it can eat with less danger from predators.

Chipmunks eat a lot in autumn. They have to eat enough food to keep their bodies nourished throughout winter, because they hibernate in an underground burrow from October until April, while snow covers the ground in the mountains.

There are four species of chipmunk in BC. The species that lives on Dog Mountain is the yellow-pine chipmunk, formerly called the northwestern chipmunk. Chipmunks belong to the same family (Sciuridae) as squirrels. Chipmunks are smaller than squirrels and have distinctive light and dark stripes running along their backs and faces. At lower elevations you might see Townsend's Chipmunk *(Tamias townsendii)*.

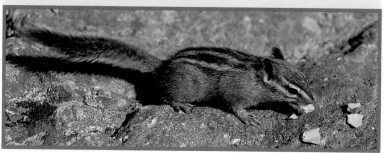

Continue along the rocky and root-tangled trail for another 25 to 30 minutes. Soon you will see First Lake. In the early part of summer there are lots of flying insects here, including mosquitoes, flies and other species that don't bite, such as dragonflies. By September, though, it is usually too cool here for most bugs to survive. Stop for a rest and have something to drink.

The trail passes some smaller ponds, then it's back to the forest. There's lots to see on the forest floor: ferns, shrubs, mosses and more.

Stay on the trail for another 30 to 40 minutes, until you reach some big rock outcrops. Where the trail forks, go left. Go past a big hemlock tree to emerge onto some big rock bluffs, also known as Dog Mountain.

Find a safe place to sit to enjoy all the great views. There are mountains to the north and the city to the south. If you open up your lunch, you'll probably get some mountain visitors (see p. 63 and below).

When you've finished lunch, explore around the south (city) side of the rock bluffs to find some old logs and rusted bits of metal (see p. 65).

When you're ready to go, return the same way you came. Be sure that you go right at the sign, toward the parking lot.

Grey Jay *(Perisoreus canadensis)*

Also known as whiskey jack, camp robber and Canada jay, this pretty grey and white bird is in the same bird family as crows and ravens. Like those birds, it is very intelligent.

Grey jays eat mostly insects and fruit—and sometimes carrion (dead animals). But they're also happy to share any nuts or fruit lurking in your lunch. To ensure that they have something to eat during winter, grey jays paste little balls of food scraps together with saliva (spit) and hang them among conifer needles.

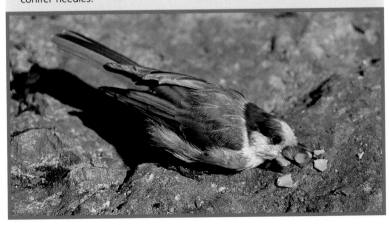

The Lookout Cabins

These logs and metal bits are all that is left of two cabins that were used as forest-fire lookouts by workers of the Greater Vancouver Water District. These lookout posts are no longer needed because observers in airplanes and pictures from satellites can provide better information about any fires that might be burning in the forest.

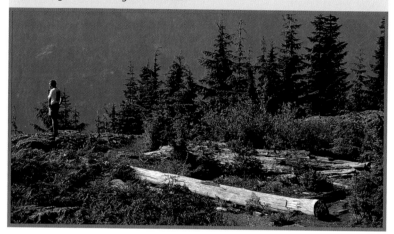

View from Dog Mountain

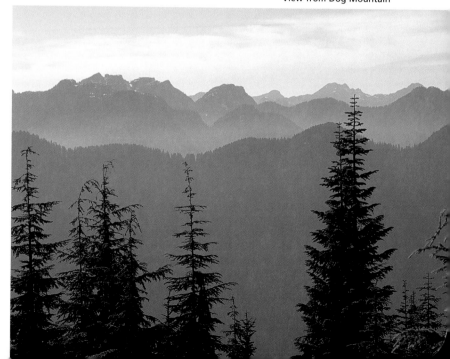

Goldie and Flower Lakes

Length: 3.5-km loop

Time needed: 1.5 to 2 hours

Season: July to September

Rating: Moderate

Dogs: Yes, on leash

Stroller-friendly: No

Washrooms: At parking lot

Highlights: Subalpine lakes, subalpine plants, insects, golden-crowned kinglet

Access: Follow Highway 1 (Upper Levels Highway) to just north of the Second Narrows Bridge, and take the exit for Mount Seymour and Lillooet Road. Keep right to get onto Mount Seymour Parkway and head eastward. At Parkgate Centre, turn left onto Mount Seymour Road and follow it to the large parking area at the very top.

Driving time: 45 minutes

Mount Seymour Provincial Park has long been a popular destination for hikers. Although most hikers head for the heights of Mount Seymour or the bluffs of Dog Mountain (p. 62), there's also this pretty little loop through classic subalpine forest and past tiny jewel-like lakes.

From the parking area, find the first-aid building (marked with a red cross on a white triangle). On the right of the building there is a dirt road with a sign pointing the way to Goldie Lake. Follow the wide path past the rope-tow building and down the ski trail.

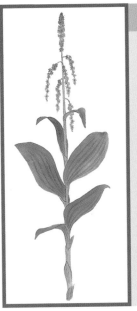

Goldie Lake

Like most subalpine lakes, Goldie Lake is surrounded by a marshy shoreline. Species of plants that you might not see elsewhere grow here. Look for Indian hellebore (shown in illustration), twistedstalk (a medium-sized plant with oval leaves and tiny, bell-shaped, greenish flowers) and mountain-heather (a short plant with tiny, needle-like leaves and pink or purple flowers).

Aside from the flowery plants that grow here, there are also less showy plants, including the sedges. Sedges are related to grasses and rushes. In fact, it can be pretty tough to tell a grass from a rush or a sedge. The easiest way to tell them apart is to remember this little rhyme about their stems: 'Sedges have edges, rushes are round, grasses are hollow, where willows abound.'

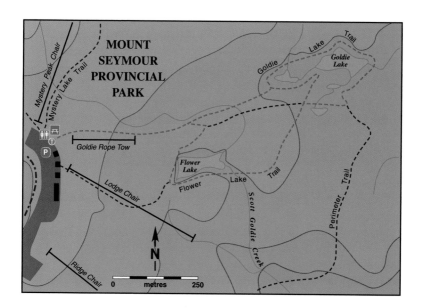

At the bottom of the hill, look on the right for a gravel path—the beginning of the Goldie Lake Trail—that heads into the trees. It's marked with the familiar square orange trail markers. A few minutes later you will reach a junction with the Flower Lake Trail. Go left to continue on the Goldie Lake Trail, past stunted, twisted trees and blueberry shrubs. Cross a small wooden bridge and, a bit farther, a second bridge over Scott-Goldie Creek.

The Subalpine

As the name suggests, the subalpine zone is just below the alpine zone. But what do these terms actually mean?

The alpine zone is the part of a mountain that is above the treeline; the highest elevation where trees don't grow and the biggest plants are small, shrub-like clumps. The subalpine zone consists of the forests and meadows that are just below the treeline. Trees, shrubs and many other plants grow here, but they are much smaller than they would be if they grew in forests or meadows at lower elevations.

The cold and snow of the subalpine mean that plants have a shorter growing season; there are fewer days when the snow is gone and temperatures are high enough for a plant to grow.

The elevations where alpine zones and subalpine zones occur varies. In the warmer southwestern corner of the province, the treeline can be as high as 1675 metres. In the far north the treeline can start at 450 metres.

The trail descends, and, in about 15 minutes, you will arrive at the western end of Goldie Lake. At the junction you need to decide whether to go right and along the southern shore of the lake, or whether to go left for a slightly longer loop of the lake.

Whichever way you go around Goldie Lake, you will eventually come to a trail junction at its eastern end. Head south (if you took the shorter trip, that means a right turn; if you took the longer loop around, it means going left) to follow the trail to Flower Lake.

Notice the small, twisted trees on either side of the trail. They're typical of trees that grow in the subalpine.

Not much farther along there is another small subalpine lake. And, if you turn around and look behind you, you can see some steep-walled bluffs to the north. At the next trail junction, go straight to continue on the Flower Lake Trail, passing yet another small lake. Even if you haven't seen many other hikers on the trail, most summers you're guaranteed to have company by this point—in the form of hundreds of bugs.

Goldie Lake Trail

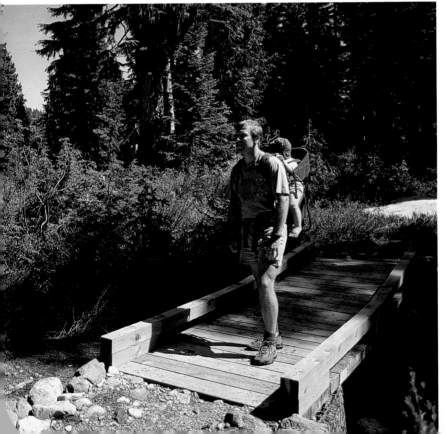

Insects of the Subalpine

Insects, especially the flying kind—flies, mosquitoes, gnats—are part of the subalpine ecosystem, like it or not. Although they may be pesky for hikers, these bugs are an important part of the food chain here.

If there weren't any insects, there would be many fewer fish, frogs, birds and other animals. That's because insects are an important food source. Creatures that you might see here that eat a lot of insects include dragonflies and swallows.

The trail climbs gently along a rocky, rooty part, then descends just as gently again. Aside from insects, there are other wild inhabitants in this part of the forest, most notably birds. Some, such as the raven and the grey jay, are easy to spot. But others—such as the golden-crowned kinglet—are more often heard than seen. Listen for their *tsee-tsee-tsee*.

The trail soon bends left to another little lake. Cross the bridge and pass a nice big yellow-cedar. Traipse along the boardwalk and head toward the sound of the creek. After you've crossed the log bridge, be sure to notice the old cabin on the left.

The trail soon leads to Flower Lake—not as big as Goldie, but with its own quiet charm. Continue along the path as it rounds the end of the lake and meets with a ski run. Stay right, going under the ski-boundary cable and along the lakeshore.

About 15 minutes later you will reach a junction. Go left. A couple of minutes later you will arrive at the junction you passed on the way in. Go left to return to the parking area—a 10- to 15-minute uphill walk.

Golden-crowned Kinglet *(Regulus satrapa)*

The Golden-crowned Kinglet is one of the tinier birds seen in these forests. In fact, they're similar in size to hummingbirds, but without the long beak. This bird has an olive green back and a dusky-white belly. Its eyes look like tiny black buttons, with a white 'eyebrow' above each. And, as the

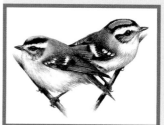

name suggests, it has a golden 'crown'—the female's crown is yellow, the male's is yellow with a reddish-orange centre.

Kinglets spend a lot of time in the trees, hopping from limb to limb, flicking their wings. Most of their time is spent foraging for food, which includes insects, spiders, fruit and seeds. They also drink tree sap.

Grey Rock

Length: 4 km

Time needed: 2 to 2.5 hours

Season: Year-round

Rating: Tough; elevation gain of 100 metres—best for ages eight and older

Dogs: Yes, on leash

Stroller-friendly: No

Washrooms: At Panorama Park

Highlights: Cedar roots, views, woodpecker holes, shore pine

Access: Take Highway 1 (Upper Levels Highway) to the north end of the Second Narrows Bridge and take the first eastbound exit. Follow Dollarton Highway to Deep Cove. At Panorama Drive, go left. Park on the right in the lot at Panorama Park.

Driving time: 30 minutes

The hike to Grey Rock can be steep for little legs that aren't used to hiking, but the sights along the way and the views at the end are the rewards for all that effort—and it's almost all downhill on the way back.

Redcedar Roots *(Thuja plicata)*

Four western redcedars have grown on top of a fallen tree that has become a 'nurse log.' As the nurse log crumbles, the roots become more and more exposed. You can see how some roots have burrowed into the ground, but they don't go all that far. Cedar trees have roots that don't grow very deep into the ground, but they do grow far outward—sometimes even farther outward than the tree is high.

Roots absorb water and minerals from the soil and pass them on to the rest of the tree. Also, they anchor the tree to keep it upright. The roots also help to hold the soil together, so that it won't be so easily washed away by rain.

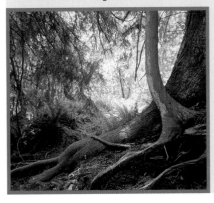

Because redcedar trees have shallow roots, the trees grow wider, as they grow older and taller. This shape gives them more stability than if they grew tall and skinny. Other species (such as the Douglas-fir) can grow much taller than the redcedar because they have roots that go deeper and cling to more soil, thereby better stabilizing the weight of the tree above.

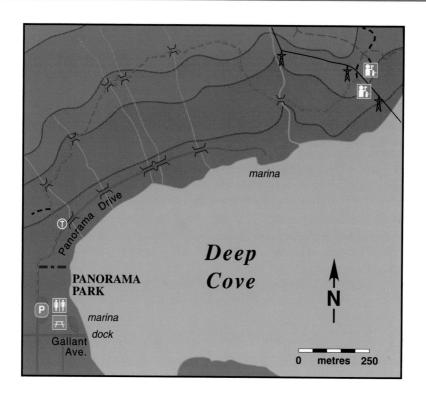

From Panorama Park, walk farther along Panorama Drive until you see the house marked 2501 Panorama. Head up the driveway to the trail-head, where a sign marks the start of the Baden-Powell Trail. (The other end of the 48-kilometre Baden-Powell Trail is at Horseshoe Bay. It was built in 1971 by 1000 Boy Scouts and Girl Guides, and it is named after the man who founded the Boy Scouts, Robert Stephenson Smyth, Lord Baden-Powell.)

The trail heads steeply uphill. Where the path widens, it also becomes rocky and rooty. Look on the left for a big tangle of tree roots (see p. 70). Stop here to catch your breath.

As you continue up the trail, there are more nurse logs and nurse stumps. Some of the tree roots clinging to the stumps look like the tentacles of an octopus. Soon you come to a boardwalk and then a bridge that crosses Panorama Creek. A few minutes later, the trail levels briefly before descending to Kia Creek.

Another few minutes brings another creek crossing. A little farther along, the trail descends into a deep ravine and crosses Cove Creek. As you come up the other side of the ravine and turn a corner, you will be greeted by a big nurse stump with a huckleberry bush growing on top. The stump is riddled with lots of holes made by woodpeckers (see p. 73).

Continue to another creek crossing. Just before the bridge there is a great big Douglas-fir. How big? About 3.5 metres in diameter—big enough that it would take at least two tall men to wrap their arms around its base.

The trail meanders a bit before dropping into another ravine and over another small creek, then climbs up the other side via a steep staircase. A few minutes later, you will cross under some power lines and descend again via switchbacks to a long boardwalk bridge over Frances Creek. Another big Douglas-fir is a bit farther ahead. The trail climbs back up, then levels off until finally you come to a junction with signs and a map.

Go right and pretty soon you will arrive at a big rock bluff—Grey Rock. It is a splendid place for a lunch break and has great views.

Before you leave Grey Rock, take a look around at the various plants that grow here. In summer, many wildflowers bloom and little white bells hang from the salal.

When you've had a good look around, a welcome rest for your feet and maybe some lunch, just retrace your steps back to Panorama Park. And remember, it's almost all downhill.

The Views from Grey Rock

Scanning from the right you can see Deep Cove with its marinas and waterfront houses. A little to the left is Indian Arm, with Burrard Inlet and Burnaby a bit farther back. If it's a clear day you can even see the tall trees of Central Park and the highrise towers of Metrotown in the distance. Almost straight across are Belcarra and its two nearby islands, Hamber and Boulder. Farther to the left is Diez Vistas Ridge, with Eagle Ridge just behind (Buntzen Lake is tucked between them, out of sight).

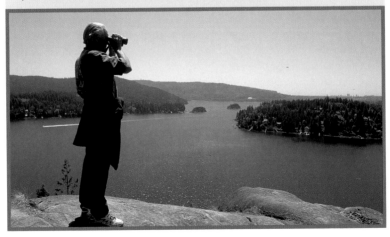

Woodpecker Holes

Using their hard, sharp bills and powerful neck muscles, woodpeckers hammer away at trees—both living and dead—in search of insects. They eat ants, beetles, caterpillars and larvae or grubs.

If you see a woodpecker hammering away on a tree, you might notice that every once in a while it stops and seems to be listening to something. In fact, woodpeckers can hear a grub munching away on the inside of a tree. And they use that noise as a guide.

You may see seven species of woodpeckers in the Lower Mainland. Some species, such as the downy woodpecker (about 17 centimetres long), are about the same size as a sparrow; others, such as the pileated woodpecker (about 43 centimetres long; see p. 175), are about the same size as a crow.

Shore Pine (*Pinus contorta* var. *contorta*)

There are only a few places on the Lower Mainland where you can see shore pine; Grey Rock is one of them. Others include Lighthouse Park in West Vancouver (p. 74), Richmond Nature Park (p. 136), Deas Island (p. 140) and Burns Bog (p. 158).

Shore pine and lodgepole pine (*Pinus contorta* var. *latifolia*) are different varieties of the same tree species. Lodgepole pine is found growing farther inland, but looking at the details—such as the two-needle bundles, pine cones and scaly bark—the two varieties appear almost identical.

So, what's the difference? Well, shore pines often have crooked, twisted (or contorted) trunks. Because of those twisty trunks, they also tend to be

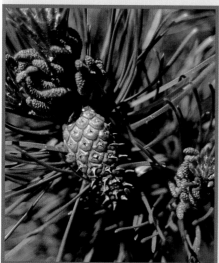

short, with the biggest of shore pines reaching a height of just 20 metres. In comparison, a lodgepole pine usually has a straight trunk and can reach 40 metres in height. The lodgepole pine also tends to have bark that is a bit redder than the shore pine's.

One of the reasons shore pine grows all crooked is that many nutrients aren't available to the tree in the habitats where it grows. As well, shore pine trees often have to deal with a lot of salt, which slows their growth.

Lighthouse Park

Length: 2.5-km loop

Time needed: 1.5 to 2 hours

Season: Year-round

Rating: Moderate; lots of ups and downs over rocky and rooty terrain

Dogs: Yes, on leash

Stroller-friendly: All-terrain stroller, if you're willing to carry it at times

Washrooms: Outhouses on trail near starting point; at cabin near lighthouse; and across road from Douglas-fir cross-section

Highlights: Douglas-fir, ancient rocks, lighthouse, tree rings

Access: Follow Marine Drive westward through West Vancouver, past Caulfeild Cove. Turn left onto Beacon Lane, at the Lighthouse Park sign; follow the road to the right and park in the lot.

Driving time: 40 minutes

Lighthouse Park is unique in the Lower Mainland because it is low-level old-growth forest that has never been logged. (Even Stanley Park's forests have seen some logging.) Here you can see an example of what all of the Lower Mainland's forests once looked like, and you can learn how an old-growth forest ecosystem functions.

View from Lighthouse Park

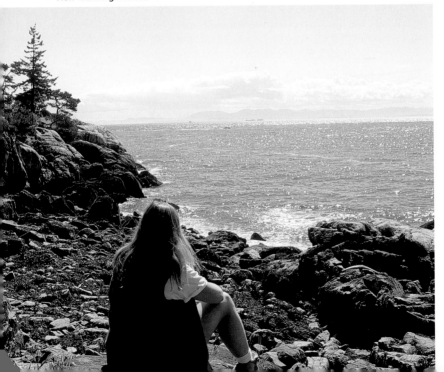

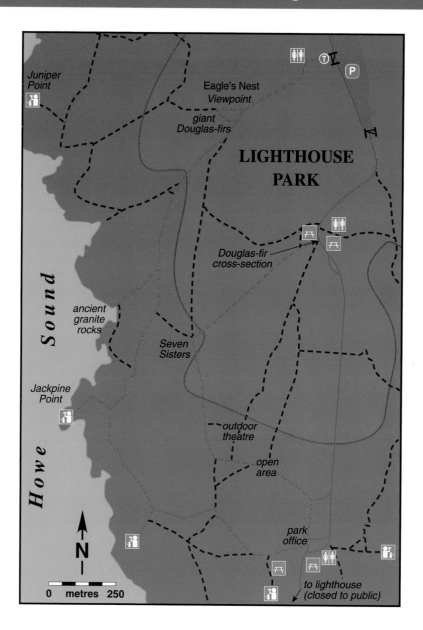

The hike's starting point is the yellow gate about halfway up the parking area. Head west (past a couple of outhouses) along a wide path. Almost immediately you will have big trees all around you. Most of these giants are Douglas-firs.

You will come to a junction with the trail to Juniper Point. You'll continue left, but it's worth a short wander to the right to see three Douglas-fir giants.

Return to the main trail and go right where there is a western redcedar root that looks like a long leg meant to trip unsuspecting hikers. In fact, as a sign above it says, the leg is actually a 'hanging-in-mid-air root' that shows that this tree didn't grow directly from the ground, but from a nurse log, now long gone. (The word 'nurse' comes from a Latin word that means 'to nourish.' Nurse logs are trees that have fallen down. In places where the soil may be thin or poor, they provide seedling trees with nutrients and a good place to grow.)

A bit farther along, stay to the right of some fencing that was put there to help a part of the forest recover from erosion. Ignore the secondary trail on the right and continue past more big Douglas-firs. One has a branch high up that makes it look like a weightlifter flexing his muscles.

Where the next secondary trail branches toward the water, go right to a rocky viewpoint—a great place to watch the sea, the sea birds and the waves.

Retrace your steps to the main trail and go right (south). A few minutes later, a side trail hooks sharply right to Jackpine Point. Here, among the gnarled arbutus, are the 'jackpine' that give the point its name.

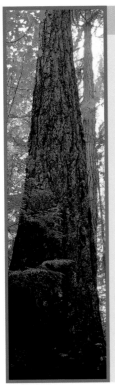

Douglas-fir *(Pseudotsuga menziesii)*

The Douglas-fir can grow taller than any other species of tree native to Canada. Most of the Douglas-fir trees in Lighthouse Park stand between 55 and 60 metres tall. One on the eastern side of the park measures 77.1 metres tall.

Even though the Douglas-firs in Lighthouse Park are big, they're shorter than the largest Douglas-fir in Canada, which grows in the Coquitlam River watershed. It stands 94.3 metres tall and measures 17.3 metres around. That's as tall as some of the office buildings in downtown Vancouver.

An even taller Douglas-fir, the Brummet Fir, grows near Coos Bay, Oregon. It stands 99 metres tall and measures about 11 metres around. To get some idea of just how big this tree is, imagine how tall a 25-storey office building stands. Or imagine about 55 average-sized adult men stacked one on top of the other.

Trees this tall were rare even before commercial logging began in North America. They grew so big only in places where the soil and climate were just right, and where they were sheltered from the wind by the surrounding forest and the shape of the land.

Ancient Rocks

The salt-and-pepper rocks here are made of granite. Granite is a blend of two minerals, quartz (the 'salt') and feldspar (the 'pepper'). As the sign says, the rocks here are estimated to be about 100 million years old.

They were formed deep below the earth's surface when big blobs of magma (molten rock) cooled. Geologists use the word 'plutonic'—from Pluto, the Roman god of the underworld—to describe rocks that were formed in this way.

These plutonic rocks eventually worked their way up to where they are today as a result of geological forces such as uplift. (Uplift occurs when layers of bedrock are squashed, folded or warped.) They were then rounded off by the movement of glaciers during the various ice ages.

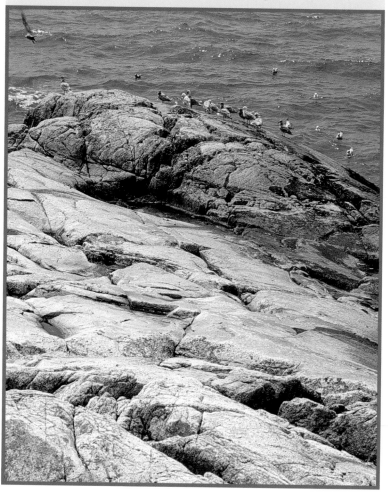

The Point Atkinson Lighthouse

The first lighthouse here—with a steam-powered foghorn—was built in 1874. Not long afterward, all the land that is now park was set aside as a reserve by the federal government. (The city of West Vancouver now leases the land from the federal government for $1 per year.) Therefore we have the building of the lighthouse to thank for this beautiful pocket of wilderness.

The original lighthouse burned down and was replaced in 1910 with the concrete lighthouse that you see today.

For generations, lighthouse keepers and their families tended the light. These days, though, the lighthouse is automated although a resident caretaker still lives in the adjoining house. To protect the caretaker's privacy, the grounds are off-limits to the public, except for most weekends when the public is allowed to pass through the gates to look at the lighthouse.

Point Atkinson Lighthouse

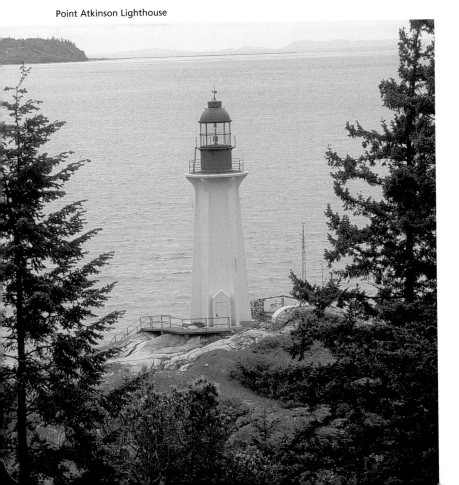

Properly known as 'shore pine' (*Pinus contorta*; see p. 73), this species is also called 'scrub pine' and 'lodgepole pine.' (This type of confusion is one reason botanists favour using scientific names.)

Return to the main trail and continue south to the next side trail, which leads to a 40-metre-high bluff of more 100-million-year-old rock. The bluff has a view of the lighthouse and is a good spot to have lunch or a snack.

Return to the main trail and follow it southward again. For a closer look at the lighthouse, as well as a cluster of old cabins, bear right just past the sign that indicates the side trail to West Beach. (One of the cabins has public washrooms.) The buildings were constructed and used during the Second World War, when the light of the lighthouse was used to watch for any enemy submarines or ships that might try to enter Burrard Inlet.

Then look just beyond the water taps and the grey building for the trail marked by yellow triangles. Follow it to an open area, staying left to pass the outdoor theatre, and, 100 metres farther, you'll meet a trail junction. Here stands a grove of Douglas-fir and western redcedar that is known as 'the Seven Sisters.' Look for the trail heading inland; it is marked by stairs and a recently toppled snag.

The paved park road soon comes into sight. Stay left and, about 10 metres from the road, stop and turn around. You should be facing a cross-section of a 525-year-old Douglas-fir (see below).

Go left on the paved road and uphill. Another 150 metres or so brings you to the upper end of the parking area. There are many other trails to explore in Lighthouse Park. Maps to help guide your way are available at the information signboard.

Tree Rings

The old Douglas-fir, which died of natural causes in 1977, would have been a seedling in the 1450s. Elsewhere at about that time, Montezuma was the head of the Aztec Empire, Gutenberg was publishing the first printing-press edition of the Bible and Christopher Columbus was still a young boy.

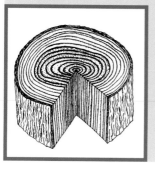

Although it would be tough to do, because of all the graffiti that has been carved into this cross-section, you could find the precise age of the tree by counting its rings and reading its life history. Each ring tells the story of one year of the tree's life: the wider rings show when a tree grew quickly, when the growing conditions were very good. The narrower rings show years of slow growth, perhaps when the tree faced a drought or an insect infestation.

Cypress Falls

Length: 3 km

Time needed: 2 to 2.5 hours

Season: Year-round

Rating: Moderate; elevation gain of 80 metres

Dogs: Yes, on leash

Stroller-friendly: No

Washrooms: None

Highlights: Waterfalls, banana slugs, Douglas-fir, nurse logs

Access: Follow Highway 1 (Upper Levels Highway) westward to the exit for Caulfeild and Woodgreen Drive. Go right on Woodgreen Drive and pass Woodcrest Road; turn right on Woodgreen Place. There are two parking areas: one, near the tennis courts, has just a few spots, but there's more parking in an old gravel pit a little farther along.

Driving time: 45 minutes

Most people know about Cypress Provincial Park, but not as many know about Cypress Falls Park, even though it's only a short distance away. Cypress Falls is a small West Vancouver municipal park with waterfalls, old-growth trees and great hiking trails.

Cypress Falls trail

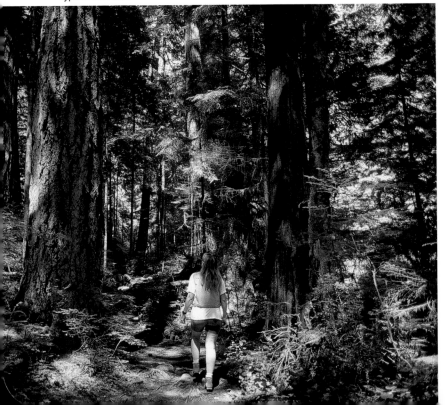

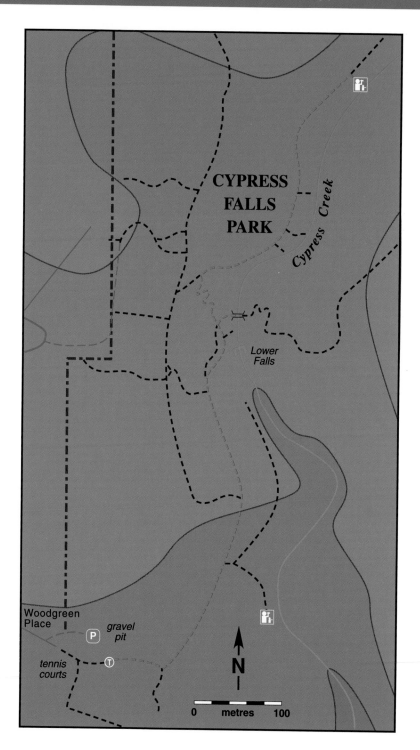

CYPRESS
FALLS
PARK

Cypress Creek

Lower
Falls

Woodgreen
Place

gravel
pit

tennis
courts

N

0   metres   100

From the parking area, head toward the trees to find the main trail. Go left and follow the trail as it climbs slowly upward. Where the path forks, go straight ahead. Even on a hot day, the air is cool here, thanks to the forest. Check out the different kinds of trees, but also be sure to watch along the trail for a certain animal that likes things cool and damp—the banana slug.

The trail will bring you to a rustic wooden bridge and Cypress Creek. Just downstream of the bridge is the Lower Falls. Take the side trail for a good view of the water as it squeezes through a narrow opening in the rocks, bounces off a rock ledge and falls to the pool below.

Retrace your steps to the main trail and continue upward and north. At the next junction, go right to stay with the main trail as it shadows Cypress Creek. You will pass through a small grove of big trees (see p. 83).

At one point, about halfway to the Upper Falls, a short side trail leads to a tiny rocky beach on Cypress Creek. This beach is a good place to take a break and maybe have lunch or a snack before continuing ahead.

The trail rolls along, in some places going up for a bit and in others going down to cross a small creek or marsh where moisture-loving trees (such as the western redcedar) grow. As you continue along the trail, you will pass many more big trees. Some trees have fallen to the forest floor. Even though they are no longer living, these trees continue to contribute to the growth of the forest (see p. 84).

Banana Slug *(Ariolimax columbianus)*

The banana slug is one of the largest slugs in the world and can grow as long as 26 centimetres—almost as long as a standard ruler. It is one of about 12 species of slugs that live in BC's forests.

Slugs are mollusks, which makes them relatives of snails, clams and oysters. Their heads have what look like four little feelers poking out. The slug's eyes are at the ends of the two longer, upward-pointing appendages, but a slug can't see like you can. A slug's eyes don't see images, but they are sensitive to changes in the amount of light.

Slugs have seven different kinds of slime that they secrete to help them move along. The strongest type of slime lets them lower themselves down tree trunks.

Banana slugs prefer to be out at night, when it's cool, dark and damp. They are big eaters. They love to gobble up the leaves and stems of plants. Banana slugs are different from the slugs that you might find in a city garden and that eat flowers and vegetables. Those urban slugs, which include the giant black slug and the great spotted slug, were accidentally imported from Europe. Some of them kill and eat our native slugs.

As you continue along the trail, keep your ears open. You might hear the chattering of a Douglas's squirrel or the knock-knock-knock of a woodpecker. You will notice that the sound of the creek is getting louder, but not because you're getting closer to it—it's because you are nearing the Upper Falls (see p. 84).

A couple of side trails head off to the right, but they don't have very good views of the falls. The side trail to the best viewpoint leaves the main trail near the top, from where you can already see the falls. For a better look, head down the side trail a short way, but stay well away from the edge—it's a long and rocky way down.

Once you've taken in the sights, just turn around and retrace your steps downhill to return to the parking area.

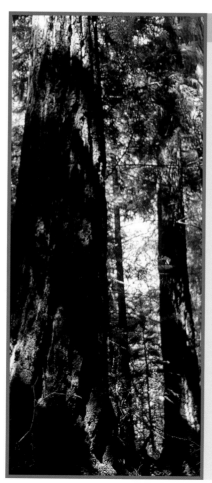

The Douglas-fir Burns

Scientists believe that these Douglas-fir trees are about 400 years old. They were seedlings when Galileo disclosed that the earth revolved around the sun and not the other way around, as was commonly believed at the time.

These trees not only escaped being cut down when most of the other trees here were logged about 70 to 80 years ago, but they also survived at least one big forest fire. You can see clues of the fire on the trunks of the trees.

Look on the lower parts for blackened bark that shows where these trees were burned by the heat and the flames. Most kinds of trees wouldn't survive such a forest fire, but the inner wood of a mature Douglas-fir tree doesn't get burned because it has bark up to 15 centimetres thick, almost as thick as a brick is long. Although Douglas-fir trees can survive a moderate forest fire, if it's a really big, really fierce fire, even they will die.

Nurse Logs

When a tree falls to the forest floor, water from the ground and from rain soak into it more easily. Twigs, leaves and needles fall onto it. Moss, lichen, fungi and bacteria begin to grow. These conditions make the fallen tree (or log) rot, but they also make the log into the perfect place for a seed to grow. In essence, the log 'nurses' the seedlings with water and nutrients.

Nurse logs are very important to the growth of new conifer trees in a rainforest, because almost all conifer seedlings grow on rotting stumps and logs. In some species, such as the western hemlock, up to 80 percent of regeneration takes places on nurse logs and stumps.

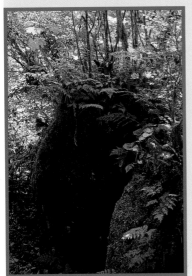

Fallen trees also serve other important functions in the forest. They can provide shelter for small mammals, insects and amphibians. They slow the runoff from rain, so that it has more time to seep into the soil, making the water more available to plants and trees and less likely to cause erosion and flooding. And, because some really big logs can take hundreds of years to break down completely, they keep passing nutrients into the soil for a long, long time.

The Upper Falls

The Upper Falls (shown in the photo, opposite) look different from the falls that you saw down below. Because there's no narrow slot for the water to squeeze through, the creek sweeps over the rock and drops 10 metres (that's taller than the height of five adults standing one on top of the other) into a pool. Then the water sweeps over more rock and drops to another pool before it straightens out and flows as a creek again.

The rock here is called quartz diorite. It's made up of quartz, feldspar and hornblende—all pretty hard minerals. It was formed between 140 and 180 million years ago, deep beneath the surface of the earth, when some magma hardened. Over time this rock was pushed upward by geological forces such as earthquakes. Meanwhile, glacial action and other forces of erosion were at work removing the overlying materials. Erosion, with help from the waters of Cypress Creek, is still at work on the rock today.

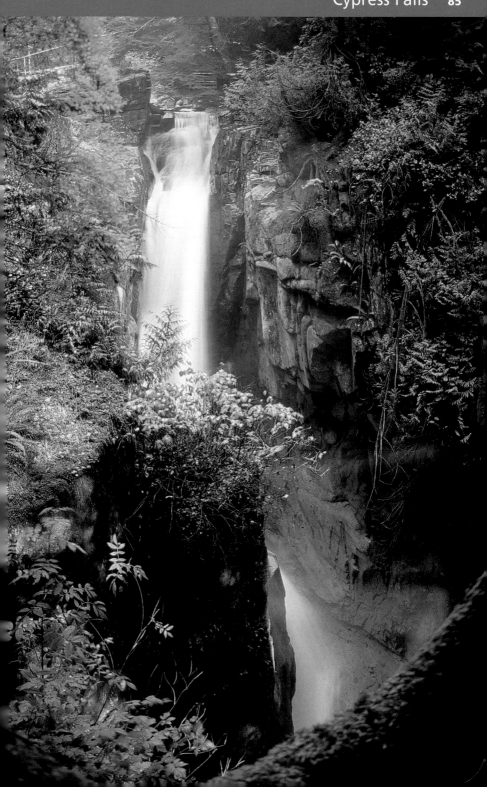

Yew Lake

Length: 2.3-km loop

Time needed: 1 to 1.5 hours

Season: June to October

Rating: Easy

Dogs: Yes, on leash

Stroller-friendly: All-terrain stroller only

Washrooms: At cafeteria; outhouses near trailhead

Highlights: Yellow-cedar, blueberries, black bears, pond-lilies

Access: Follow Highway 1 (Upper Levels Highway) to West Vancouver and take exit 8 to Cypress Provincial Park. Follow Cypress Parkway (Cypress Bowl Road) all the way to its end at the downhill ski area parking lot.

Driving time: 40 minutes

The Yew Lake Trail is probably the easiest hike into the subalpine of the North Shore mountains, and it is one of the prettiest hikes too. This flat, wide, wheelchair-accessible trail wanders through the Yew Lake meadows with its lush vegetation and old-growth trees.

From the parking area, head north, past the ski area buildings. At the northern end of the ticket building, look on the left for the signpost that points the way to the 'Yew Lake/Old Growth Loop.' Cypress Creek trickles by, first on the left, then on both sides of the trail.

Yellow-cedar *(Chamaecyparis nootkatensis)*

Yellow-cedar looks similar to western redcedar, but there are several ways to tell them apart. The easiest is to crush a few of the scale-like leaves; they have a smell that is kind of musty and unpleasant compared to the more familiar scent of western redcedar.

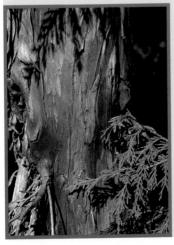

Some of the yellow-cedars in Cypress Park are more than 1100 years old, but the oldest one in this part of the park is about 850 years old.

First Nations peoples have used the yellow-cedar for all kinds of things. The wood was used to make tools, dishes, paddles, masks and chests. The bark was used to make blankets, robes, hats and capes. Shredded bark was used to make towels, washcloths and bandages.

One yellow-cedar in the Yew Lake area shows axe marks and bark-stripping scars that date from about 400 years ago.

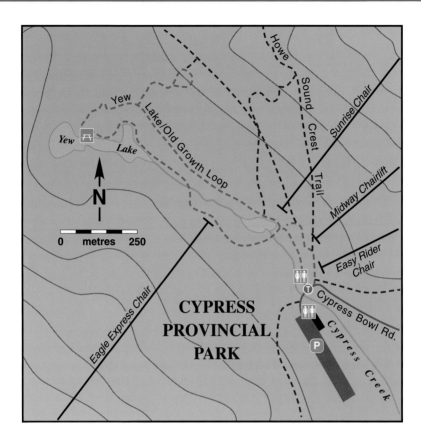

At the first trail junction, continue straight ahead to follow the path as it enters the trees. In summer, when the sun can be blazing, this section remains cool and shady. Notice the trees around you. Although they're not very big compared to some of the trees that you might see at lower elevations in places such as Lighthouse Park or Stanley Park, some of them are just as old.

Because it's colder here and because snow covers the ground for much of the year, there is only a short period of time for plants to grow. A tree in the subalpine might just have three months per year to grow, whereas trees at lower elevations might have twice as long.

One kind of tree that you'll see here is the yellow-cedar, also known as the yellow-cypress. Cypress Creek and Cypress Provincial Park were named after this tree.

You'll arrive at a second junction a few minutes after passing the first junction. Go right to walk the Old Growth Loop. It's a short loop with some really big mountain hemlock and amabilis fir trees. They range up to about 60 metres in height—as tall as some of the biggest trees in

Stanley Park and Lighthouse Park. When you consider how slowly trees grow at this elevation, their size is even more remarkable.

When you've returned to the start of the loop, go right and retrace your steps to the junction where you left the Yew Lake Trail. Go right again here. The trail soon enters Yew Lake meadows—wetlands that were formed a long time ago when glaciers dug a deep depression here. At first the depression filled with meltwater. Eventually plants grew, died and were compacted, forming a layer of peat.

Not all plants flourish in these kinds of conditions, but many species of blueberries do very well here.

If you're here in late summer or early autumn, be sure to sample some blueberries. But also be sure to keep a lookout for black bears (see p. 89). They also love to eat the blueberries and you can often see bears hunkered down among the bushes, gobbling berries.

The trail continues and you soon reach Yew Lake, which is a good place to stop for lunch or a snack—if there aren't too many bugs, that is. The water is shallow and is usually filled with various kinds of vegetation, including yellow pond-lilies (see p. 89).

As you continue along the trail, you soon reach the outlet end of Yew Lake, where Cypress Creek begins. The creek flows alongside the trail for a while, then you cross a small bridge over the creek. Soon you're back to the ski area. Follow the path right, past the Eagle Chair. At the next junction go left and continue on the path along the dirt road. Follow the path left as it descends into the trees. The trail takes you back to the first junction near the Sunrise Chair. Then you need only retrace your earlier steps back to the parking lot.

Blueberries *(Vaccinium* spp.)

Although they're hard to tell apart, four species of blueberries grow in this area. These wild blueberries are different from the farm-grown kind that you buy at the store, but they're still edible.

Some species of blueberry, such as oval-leaved blueberry, produce sweeter berries than other species. And in some species, such as Alaskan blueberry, you

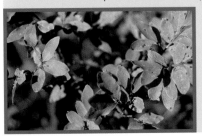

might find that certain bushes yield sweeter berries than others.

BC First Nations peoples ate blueberries in a number of different ways: fresh, dried or mixed with fish oil or animal fat. More recently, they have canned or frozen the berries or made jam with them.

Black Bear *(Ursus americanus)*

Black bears are, as the name suggests, usually black. But they can also be brown or cinnamon coloured. In some parts of BC the fur of *Ursus americanus* can be white or even 'blue'—actually a steely grey colour.

Male black bears, measured nose to tail, can be as long as a man is tall and weigh 110 to 270 kilograms. Female black bears are shorter (as long as a 10- or 12-year-old child is tall) and weigh 90 to 200 kilograms.

Black bears are omnivores—they eat all kinds of things, just like people. They eat vegetation, such as berries, roots and grasses, and they also eat animals, such as insects, fish and small mammals.

Some people who hike worry that they'll be attacked by a bear. To read about how to avoid bear encounters, see p. 15.

Yellow Pond-lily *(Nuphar polysepalum)*

Depending on the time of year that you're here, you might see lots of big yellow flowers floating on the surface of Yew Lake, or you might see just heart-shaped green leaves. What you won't see are the pond-lilies' rhizomes (pronounced 'rye-zomes') that are buried in the muck below.

Rhizomes are more like stems than roots, but they also act like roots in some ways—they anchor the plant and serve as a kind of nutrient storehouse for winter months. Yellow pond-lily rhizomes can grow to 5 metres long.

Lots of creatures depend on yellow pond-lilies for food and shelter. Dragonflies and damselflies rest on the lilies, as do frogs and ducklings. Other animals, including some beetles, snails and frogs, lay their eggs on the undersides of the leaves.

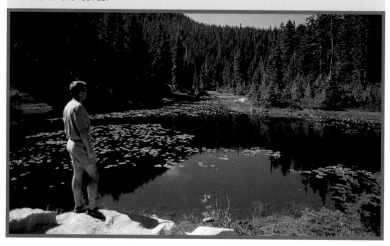

Hollyburn Ridge

Length: 3.5-km loop

Time needed: 2 to 2.5 hours

Season: June to October

Rating: Moderate

Dogs: Yes, on leash

Stroller-friendly: All-terrain stroller only

Washrooms: Outhouses at parking area and near warming hut

Highlights: Heritage cabins, mountain hemlock, subalpine lakes, subalpine insects, heather

Access: Follow Highway 1 (Upper Levels Highway) to West Vancouver and take exit 8 to Cypress Provincial Park. Follow Cypress Parkway (Cypress Bowl Road) and take the turn-off to the right to the cross-country ski area parking lot.

Driving time: 40 minutes

This hike follows trails that have been used by hikers and skiers since the 1920s and 1930s. Along the way are some of the old cabins and lifts that were used by the skiers of that era. There are also very old trees, small lakes and plants that only grow in the mountains.

From the trailhead sign, follow the wide path toward the forest and the Hollyburn Lodge sign. If you're hiking here in summer, you'll see

The Old Cabins

During the 1920s, 30s and 40s, hikers and skiers stayed in this old cabin and others nearby. Before the Lions Gate Bridge and the Cypress Bowl Parkway were built, hikers and skiers had to take a ferry from Vancouver to West Vancouver and then walk all the way uphill. These days, people just drive back and forth from home, and the cabins stand unused.

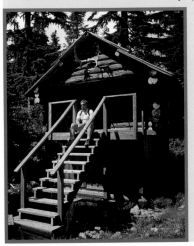

Continue past more cabins toward the red building just ahead—Hollyburn Lodge. It was built in 1926 from lumber salvaged from a dismantled mill that used to be farther down the mountain. In winter it's still used by cross-country skiers and snowshoers as a warm, cozy place to take a lunch break. In summer and autumn the lodge is closed, but there are picnic tables tucked behind the blueberry bushes where you can stop for a snack or lunch.

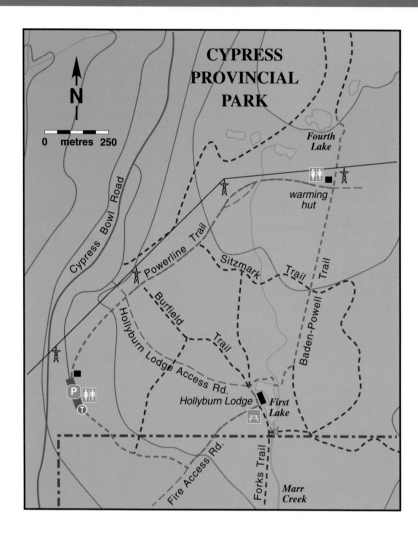

wildflowers—such as purple lupine, red fireweed and white valerian—on both sides of the path. By autumn the flowers are mostly gone, but you'll see purple-blue blueberries dangling from bushes everywhere. They're edible, but don't eat too many, because the birds, bears and other animals that live here need them.

Within 10 to 15 minutes you reach a junction. Stay right. Not much farther along, there's an old ski cabin adorned with antlers. The front of the lodge looks out onto First Lake, a small subalpine lake (or 'tarn'). Continue along the shore past the ranger station and over a little bridge. A few metres farther along you reach a four-way junction with a signpost and map. Go left.

As you go up the little rise, take a look at the trees on the left. You won't see this species of tree much farther down the mountain. Here on the south coast it grows only in the elevation range of 750 to 1800 metres. (We're at about 925 metres elevation here.) This tree is the mountain hemlock.

Continue straight ahead to a viewpoint that overlooks First Lake and Hollyburn Lodge. Just behind you, hidden in the bushes, is an old ski-lift engine. Follow the path downhill to an intersection with the Sitzmark Trail. Continue straight ahead, this time climbing uphill and following the signs for the warming hut.

Just where there is a rocky outcrop and the trail levels off, look for an old stump on the left. Look at how closely spaced its tree rings are. This tree was probably about 700 to 800 years old when it was cut.

Farther up the trail is the warming hut—a wood cabin used in winter by cross-country skiers as a warm place to take a break. Go past the hut a bit farther to Fourth Lake, the biggest of four little lakes nearby.

The lake is small but beautiful. One of the first things that you'll probably notice is that it's also very popular with bugs. Although some of the

Mountain Hemlock *(Tsuga mertensiana)*

Two species of hemlock tree are found in BC: the western hemlock and the mountain hemlock. Since the western hemlock can grow from sea level to 1500 metres in elevation, there is an overlap of 750 metres in their elevation ranges and you need other ways to tell them apart.

So, what clues can help you recognize a mountain hemlock other than its elevation range? Look on the forest floor beneath the tree that you are trying to identify for cones that have fallen from it. Mountain hemlock cones

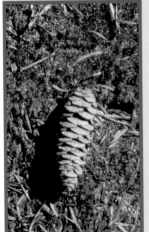

(shown in photo) are shaped like miniature corn cobs. They can be as long as an adult's finger. Western hemlock cones are roundish and smaller, about the size of a grape.

You can also look at the tree's needles. If a needle has two white bands on the underside, then the tree is a western hemlock. If not, it's mountain hemlock.

Sometimes, though, you'll find a hemlock that can be hard to identify as being one species or the other. It might have some clues that make you think it's a western hemlock and others that make you think it's a mountain hemlock. Then you know that you have found a hybrid (blend) of both types, which sometimes happens.

Pink Mountain-Heather
(Phyllodoce empetriformis)

Like many plants that grow in the subalpine, pink mountain-heather never grows very large. The biggest that pink mountain-heather ever gets is about 40 centimetres in height (about the length of a sheet of legal-sized paper).

They don't get very big because they grow high in the mountains, where snow can last well into June or July. Plants at lower elevations can start growing much earlier. Come October, temperatures in the subalpine drop to freezing and snow starts falling again. Mountain plants get a shorter time to grow, bloom and produce seeds than lowland plants do.

The short growing season is also why you should stick to the trails when hiking in the mountains. Plants such as mountain-heather take a long time to recover once damaged.

insects that hang around here aren't very pleasant (such as mosquitoes and some biting flies) there is at least one kind of insect that won't annoy you and is lots of fun to watch: the water strider.

Retrace your steps to the warming hut and go right (west) along the Powerline Trail. There are more lakes on the right and gnarled mountain hemlocks. In summer, look on the side of the trail for clusters of tiny, bell-like, purple-pink flowers: they are pink mountain-heather.

Continue along the Powerline Trail to the top of a big downhill slope. As you head down the slope to the parking area, enjoy the beautiful views (weather permitting) of Point Grey, Vancouver, Georgia Strait and many of the Gulf and San Juan islands.

Water Striders (Family Gerridae)

Water striders, also known as pond skaters, are small, from dime-sized to nickel-sized, if you include the legs. The front pair of legs is used to grab prey, the middle pair is used to paddle and the back pair is used to steer.

Water striders scoot along the surface of the water much as ice skaters move on ice. Lots of fine little hairs on their feet let them literally walk on

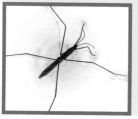

water. These hairs support the insect by distributing its weight over a greater surface area, in much the same way that snowshoes stop winter hikers from sinking into the snow.

Water striders eat small bugs that fall onto the water and get trapped on the surface or that float up from below (for example, mosquito larvae).

Killarney Lake

Length: 4.5-km loop

Time needed: 2 to 2.5 hours

Season: Year-round

Rating: Easy

Dogs: Yes, on leash

Stroller-friendly: All-terrain stroller only

Washrooms: At ferry terminals; outhouses at Killarney Lake picnic area

Highlights: Bigleaf maple, fish ladder, old cedars, dam

Access: Take Highway 1 (Upper Levels Highway) west to Horseshoe Bay. Park in the pay-parking area near the ferry terminal. (Or take a West Vancouver Blue Bus to Horseshoe Bay to avoid parking headaches.) Buy a ticket at the foot passenger booth and hop on board the Bowen Island ferry to Snug Cove—a 20-minute ride. Contact BC Ferries for sailing times and fares (see p. 248).

Driving Time: 1 hour (including the 20-minute ferry ride)

Although it's only 15 kilometres from downtown Vancouver, Bowen Island feels like a real getaway. The ferry ride to the island provides great views of Howe Sound's islands and distant peaks. The island itself feels cozy and it's the perfect place for a walk through forest and meadow, along creek and lakeshore.

Once you arrive at the Snug Cove terminal, head up Government Road to the first cross-street, Gardena Drive. Cross Government Road and pass the old Union Steamship Company Store—now home to the post office and Greater Vancouver Regional District (GVRD) offices.

About 100 metres north of the old store is a green and yellow GVRD parks sign that marks the start of the trail to Killarney Lake. Follow the trail for about 100 metres to a side trail. Go right to a small knoll with great views of the mountains.

After a look, return directly to the main trail or take a short diversion through the Bowen Memorial Garden. Either way, you emerge at a three-way junction. Take the rightmost trail to continue toward Killarney Lake.

Salmonberry bushes, ferns and old stumps line the trail. In autumn the path is covered with a thick layer of fallen leaves from the alder and maple trees (see p. 97) that tower overhead.

Hike for a few more minutes to meet a side trail on the right that leads to a viewpoint from which you can see Bridal Veil Falls. In winter and spring the falls can be quite spectacular. In summer and autumn, though, when water levels are low, the water flow is barely a trickle.

Return to the main trail and continue for 25 metres to another side trail, this one leading down to the creekside. In addition to taking you closer to the falls, this trail leads to an interesting feature: a fish ladder (see p. 97).

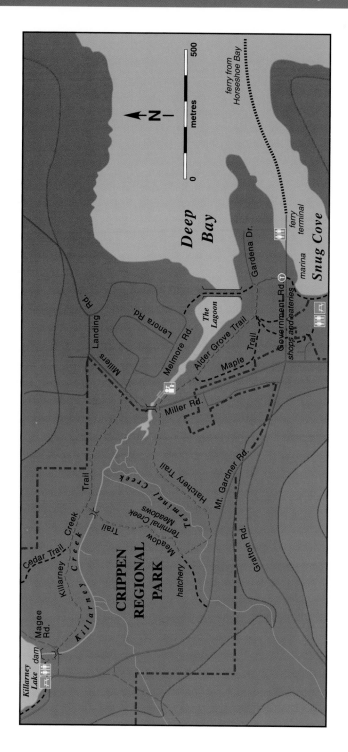

Redcedar Snags

These trees are now dead—you can see where they've been burned out from the inside. But, about 100 years ago, there were lots of western redcedar trees around here that were this big. Some were as big as 7 metres around. To get some idea of how big that is, imagine seven children in a circle with their arms outstretched, touching fingertip to fingertip.

Most of the trees in this area were logged in the 1890s and 1900s. Western redcedar was at that time used mainly for things such as shakes and shingles for houses. Redcedar is still used for shakes and shingles, and also for a lot of other things, such as fences, trellises, flower-boxes, decking, siding and panelling.

The forest here has grown back and each year the young redcedars get a little bigger, but it will take a long time—about 400 years—before any of the younger trees get as big as these snags.

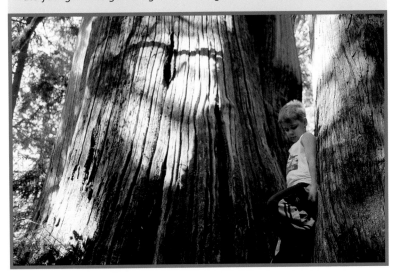

Return to the main trail and continue to the right. When you reach Miller Road, cross it and look for the green and yellow sign that points the way to Killarney Lake via the meadows and the hatchery. A short distance farther along, the trail forks. Stay right.

The forest floor is lush with sword ferns and western redcedars. You will soon come to a small footbridge. Cross the bridge and look to the right to find two huge western redcedar snags (above).

Continue on the main trail. You will descend some steps, then cross a bridge over Terminal Creek and come to the end of the Hatchery Trail. You can head left here for a short side trip to the hatchery.

Bigleaf Maple *(Acer macrophyllum)*

Bigleaf maple leaves are easy to identify—they're the same shape as the maple leaf on the Canadian flag. It's also easy to see where the bigleaf maple gets its name: some of its leaves can be as big across as a dinner plate.

Another thing you may notice about the maples here is all the moss and lichen growing on them. The moss layers may get so thick, they form a kind of soil that lets other plants—even small trees—grow on them.

First Nations peoples used many parts of the maple tree. They sometimes used the leaves to wrap food in, either to store the food temporarily or to steam it. They also used the wood to make canoe paddles and food bowls and other household implements.

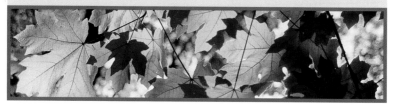

The Terminal Creek Hatchery raises about 15,000 salmon from eggs each year. After hatching and growing into fry (young fish), the salmon are ready for release. On the second Sunday of every June, schoolchildren help release all those little salmon into the creek.

Because the hatchery is run by volunteers, the opening times vary. Call (604) 947-0072 to find out when the hatchery is open or to arrange a tour for a group.

The Killarney Creek Fish Ladder

Two species of salmon are found in Killarney Creek: coho (illustrated) and chum. The chum salmon return between mid-November and early December to spawn in the gravel beds at the base of the waterfall. But the coho salmon spawn in gravel farther upstream in Killarney Creek and in Terminal Creek, so they need this fish ladder to help them get past the falls.

Once there were many more salmon in both creeks than there are today. The ladder was built in 1984 and a hatchery was established upstream to

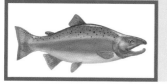

help restore the salmon stocks. In 1999 about 200 chum salmon and 100 coho salmon returned to spawn. These numbers are a long way from what they used to be, but it's the best return seen in recent years.

Return to the junction and continue straight, past the equestrian ring and through the meadows.

The trail then runs on top of an alder-lined dyke through a marshy section and over a bridge that crosses Killarney Creek. Soon you'll be at a T junction with the Killarney Creek Trail. Go left to continue to the lake. (Or, if you have had enough, you can go right to return to Snug Cove.)

A short distance farther, the Killarney Creek Trail forks. Go left to follow the signs to the Killarney Lake picnic area. About a 10- to 15-minute walk through second-growth forest will bring you to a gravel road (Magee Road). Go left and down the hill for 25 metres or so. Look on the right for the sign and trail for the picnic area.

You will emerge from the forest at the shore of the lake, which is covered with lily pads and ducks in summer. You'll also notice a small dam.

Families with older children could bear left to walk part or all of the trail that circles the lake. But those with younger kids will likely want to rest and take in the sights. Return the way you came until you reach the junction with the Meadows Trail. Then continue straight along the Killarney Creek Trail. When you reach Miller Road, cross and go about 100 metres to the right. Look for the Alder Grove Trail on the left and follow it back to Snug Cove.

Killarney Lake & Dam

Killarney Lake is relatively shallow, with lots of marshy areas that provide food and shelter for fish, birds (such as the mallard, illustrated) and other wildlife. Before the dam was built, the lake was even shallower than it is now.

The dam was built in the 1920s to ensure a constant supply of drinking water for the island. During the 1920s and 30s, much of what is now Crippen Regional Park was a big resort operated by the Union Steamship

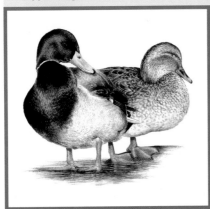

Company. There were about 180 cottages, six picnic areas, a dance pavilion that could hold 800 people and a bandshell for vaudeville shows.

The lake is no longer used as a drinking water supply, but the dam was recently fixed to keep the water level the same so that wildlife will still have the marshy areas around the lake and so that the fish habitat downstream will remain useable.

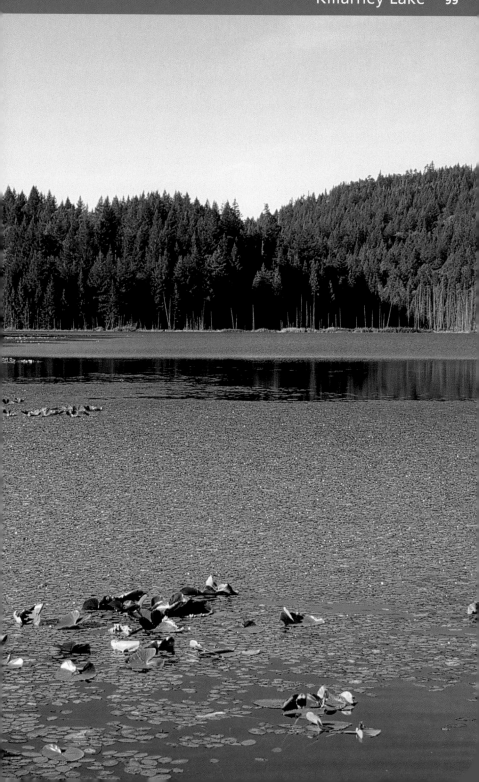

Squamish Estuary

Length: 4.5-km loop

Time needed: 2 to 2.5 hours

Season: Year-round

Note: This hike should be done only on weekends, when there is little or no industrial traffic in the area.

Rating: Easy

Dogs: Yes, on leash

Stroller-friendly: No

Washrooms: Public washrooms at Howe Sound Inn are closest.

Highlights: Mount Garibaldi, Pacific crabapple, estuary, heritage dykes

Access: Head north on Highway 99 to Squamish. At the second stoplight, turn left and follow Cleveland Avenue through downtown to Vancouver Street. Go right and park where Vancouver Street ends.

Driving time: 1 hour

Although Squamish is well known for its many mountain trails, not as many people know about the trails in one of the quieter (but equally scenic) spots, the Squamish Estuary. The estuary is important to all kinds of wildlife, from birds to butterflies and salmon to coyotes.

At the start of the hike is a map board. You can also usually find a trail brochure in the information rack at the Howe Sound Inn at the corner of Cleveland Avenue and Vancouver Street. It shows all the different trails in the estuary. This hike takes in parts of almost all the trails.

Mount Garibaldi

Mount Garibaldi is actually an old volcano. Geologists believe that it formed between 11,000 years and 15,000 years ago. It started with a spectacular eruption that spewed great clouds of ash into the air and red-hot lava onto a glacier that filled the Squamish Valley at the time. That sheet of ice was about 1350 metres thick, and only the tallest of mountains would have poked through.

Subsequent eruptions spewed more lava, and Garibaldi took on a volcano's usual cone shape. But then the climate began to warm and the glacier began to melt. And Garibaldi, which had built itself on top of the ice, began to crumble. The entire west side of Garibaldi collapsed, sending rock landslides across the valley.

What looks like the diamond-shaped top of Mount Garibaldi, Atwell Peak, is what remains of one side of the mountain. The original mountain was much bigger. To get an idea of what it might have looked like, imagine a pyramid covering the bulk of what's there today.

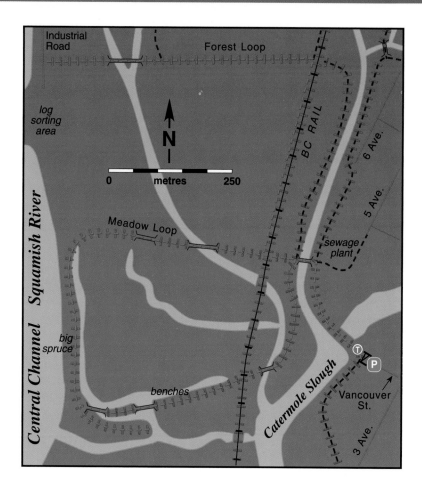

Pass through the yellow gate and go straight along the dyke. The trail crosses a slough and then curves right. This section of the trail is a good place to see birds, especially in winter when lots of ducks overwinter here.

The trail soon comes to a junction. On the right is the town's sewage plant. Go left onto a trail that leads into a copse of cottonwood and alder trees. A few minutes later, the trail emerges at the railway tracks. Cross the tracks—carefully—and go right to walk along the wide path on the west side of the tracks. (Stay clear of the tracks themselves, because trains do run here.)

As you head northward alongside the tracks, there's lots to look at, including the marshlands on both sides, wildflowers in summer and, no matter what time of year, a glorious view of Mount Garibaldi.

About a 10-minute walk or 400 metres from where you started along-side the tracks, look on the left for some pink tape fluttering from a tree branch and for a silver-coloured tag on a western hemlock that should read 'North Loop. North Dyke Trail. Squamish Estuary.' Go left here to walk along some of the oldest dykes in the estuary (see p. 105).

Along the way there are some Sitka spruce trees, and you will get occasional views of Shannon Falls and the Stawamus Chief. A few minutes along the trail, be sure to look out for 'Lesley's Headbanger,' a tree that was just a little too low for one of the Squamish Estuary Conservation Society's volunteers. The tree is a Pacific crabapple.

As you continue along the trail, notice some of the other plants growing here: the cattails, wild roses and bitter vetch, for example. About 10 to 15 minutes from Lesley's Headbanger you will come to a junction with the north end of the Forest Loop Trail. Continue straight ahead through sweet-scented forest and over some bridges for another few minutes to emerge at a gravel road (Industrial Road).

It's worth making a slight detour to the right to check out an old donkey engine and a skid used by loggers long ago. Then backtrack along the dyke that led you here until you are back at the railway tracks. Go about 400 metres to the right to find the northern end of the Meadow Loop Trail.

Pacific Crabapple *(Malus fusca)*

The Pacific crabapple is the only apple tree native to BC. (The more familiar apple trees of the backyard and the Okanagan are cultivated imports.)

In spring the tree bears lovely-smelling white or pink blossoms. The tiny, egg-shaped apples form in summer. They're about the size of big cherries. When they first appear they're green, but then they ripen to yellow and red. Although edible, they're very tart.

Crabapples were an important food for the coastal First Nations peoples. They ate them raw, boiled them, steamed them or mashed them with berries. Today First Nations peoples still eat crabapples, either raw, cooked or made into crabapple jelly.

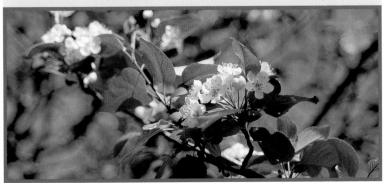

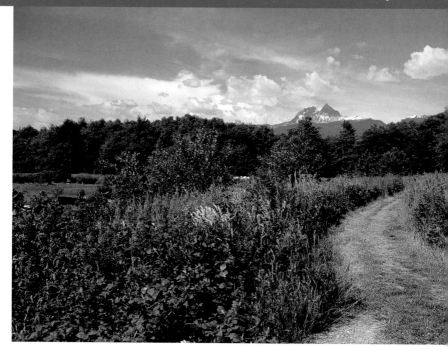

Squamish Estuary trail

The Importance of Estuaries

An estuary is the place where a river meets the sea, where fresh water meets salt water. It's also a very important place for all kinds of plants and animals.

By the time the waters of the Squamish River empty into Howe Sound, they are rich with dead and decaying plants, fish and insects. They provide food for certain plants and small animals. The plants attract herbivores, such as voles and rabbits. Small fish are eaten by bigger fish, harbour seals and great blue herons. Insects attract fish, birds and bats. Some of these animals in turn become food for larger predators: coyotes, raccoons and bears, for example.

In fact, estuaries support more kinds of plants and animals than do forests, farmland, riversides, oceans or any other type of habitat.

Although estuaries are very biologically rich, they account for less than two percent of BC's coastline. And many of those estuaries have been developed for farming, industry or housing, making them much less useful for wildlife.

Take the Squamish Estuary, for example. At one time it was much bigger, but then railways, log-sorting yards, chemical plants and ports were built on it. And there are plans to build more industrial facilities.

The Squamish Estuary Conservation Society, though, wants to preserve what's left—both for wildlife and for people. You can contact the society at Box 1274, Squamish, BC, V0N 3G0.

Go right and follow the trail through open meadow. From here you can see views all around, including Mamquam Mountain to the east, Howe Sound to the south and some of the mountains on the Sechelt Peninsula to the west. Continue along the trail as it heads toward the trees.

You will come to an alder tree with an orange diamond and a silver-coloured marker that reads 'South Loop, South Dyke Trail, Squamish Estuary.' Not much farther along you will pass a good-sized Sitka spruce. As the trail continues, the views of the Squamish River and the undyked part of the estuary open up a bit.

As the trail continues, there are more big Sitka spruce trees. One of them is about 4.5 metres around, or big enough that it would take more than three average-height adults standing fingertip to fingertip to wrap their arms around it. This tree is about 300 years old, which means that it started growing here probably even before your great-great-great-great-great-great-great-great-great-grandparents were alive.

Soon, the trail makes a sharp left. Take a break on one of the benches, where you can have a snack, look for birds or just enjoy the scenery. Then continue along the trail, which crosses the occasional bridge as it proceeds out onto the dykes.

The trail soon returns to the railway tracks. Go left. About 10 to 15 minutes of walking brings you to where you started the Meadow Loop Trail. Go right here, and, when you come to the sewage plant, go right again. Another 10 minutes and you arrive back at Vancouver Street where you started.

Squamish Estuary views

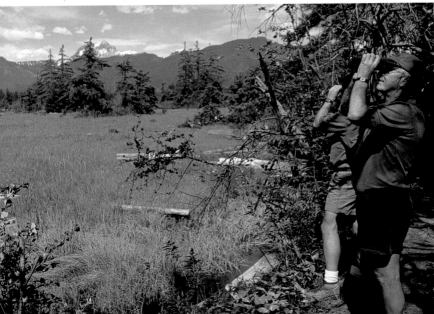

The Heritage Dykes

These dykes were built more than 100 years ago. Although they are not as old as some of the trees in this area, they're the oldest structures here that were built by people.

In the late 1880s, long before there was a road, people came from Vancouver to Squamish by steamship. Although the Squamish First Nations had lived in the area for thousands of years, it was a wild new frontier to European immigrants who were looking for a place to settle.

Some of the new settlers came to Squamish for its good agricultural land. Some people planted orchards. Others planted crops, such as hay. But at certain times of the year—in spring when the mountain snows melted, for example—the Squamish River would swell and overflow its banks. The floodwaters would cover planted fields, ruining the crops.

Around 1890 the landowners hired immigrant Chinese workers to build these dykes to keep the floodwaters out of the fields.

Hiker on heritage dyke

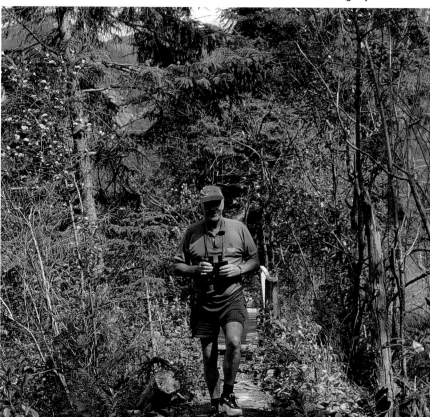

Brackendale Dykes

Length: 1.5 km

Time needed: 1 hour

Season: Year-round

Note: The best time to see lots of eagles is mid-November to mid-February.

Rating: Easy

Dogs: Yes, on leash

Stroller-friendly: All-terrain stroller only

Washrooms: Outhouse at mid-point parking area

Highlights: Bald eagles, cottonwood trees, Squamish River, salmon

Access: Follow Highway 99 north from Horseshoe Bay to Squamish. At the fourth stoplight (Garibaldi Highlands), turn left onto Garibaldi Way. At Government Road, go right. Look for the Easter Seals Camp sign on the right. Parking is available on the east side of the road, but be sure not to park on camp property.

Driving time: 1 to 1.5 hours

Even in southwestern BC, a lot of birds fly south in winter to where it's warmer, so winter is not usually the best time to see birds on a walk or hike. But the dykes at Brackendale are an exception. Come here on even the coldest days of December and January and you'll see more eagles in one place than you've ever seen before.

Bald Eagle *(Haliaeetus leucocephalus)*

Brackendale has become world famous for the number of bald eagles that come here each winter. In the winter of 1994, 3769 eagles were recorded.

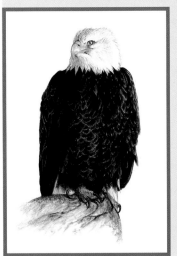

The eagles come here mostly for the food—lots of dead and dying, spawned-out salmon. In winter, to stay warm and prepare for the long flight home in spring, eagles need to eat one-tenth of their weight in food each day. That would be like an adult human eating 7 kilograms of food each day.

The eagles also come to Brackendale because there are big trees where they can rest and conserve their energy. There used to be more places in North America where eagles could overwinter, but, because of human development, there are fewer and fewer places where the birds can find food and trees and quiet.

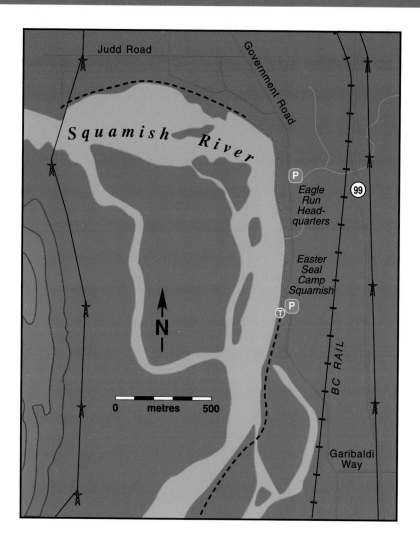

Judd Road

Government Road

S q u a m i s h   *R i v e r*

P

Eagle
Run
Head-
quarters

99

Easter
Seal
Camp
Squamish

T P

N

BC RAIL

0   metres   500

Garibaldi
Way

This hike starts from the south end of the Eagle Run dyke. There's
a wheelchair ramp that can provide good access for people with beefy
strollers, but be sure to first check that the gate is unlocked. If it is locked
you can still access the trail, but you will have to go around the gate onto
the grass.

Once you're on top of the dyke, begin scanning across the river for
eagles, especially in winter when their numbers are greater. You might
see them perched in the trees. You might see them eating salmon down
at the river's edge. You might even see them flying from place to place or,
on a clear day, soaring high above.

Continue along the dyke to a sign that tells about the First Nations heritage of the area and about what the eagles, salmon and river mean to the people native to Squamish.

As you walk toward Eagle Run headquarters, take another look across the river, but this time focus on the trees on the other side. Most of them are cottonwood trees.

You soon arrive at Eagle Run headquarters. Here there are more signs that tell more about eagles, salmon, conservation and other related topics. There are also volunteer wardens in the winter months who can answer any questions you have about the eagles. They usually have a high-power spotting scope on hand, so you can get a really close-up look at some of the eagles.

As you continue along the dyke, the Squamish River takes a wide bend toward the west. Notice the sandbars in the river—they look like little islands of sand. Each year the river changes a little bit in the direction that it flows. And each year the sandbars are a little bit different in size and in location. About the only thing that stays the same is that sandbars tend to be where the dead and dying salmon wash up.

You can continue walking along the dyke until you reach a wooden fence that marks the beginning of private property. Then just turn around and head back to where you started.

Black Cottonwood (Populus balsamifera)

The black cottonwood loves water, which is why it grows almost exclusively alongside rivers. It can grow up to 50 metres in height—taller than any other deciduous tree native to BC.

Their height is what makes cottonwood trees so attractive and important to the eagles. When they're not feeding, eagles need to rest. They don't like resting on the ground (or even in smaller trees) where they might be attacked by predators. Instead, they like to get way up high.

Sometimes the cottonwood trees here can look like eagle candelabras, with dozens of eagles in any one tree and up to 10 birds on a single branch. No one knows exactly why the eagles perch so close together, but some researchers think that they do so for additional safety, especially when they're sleeping.

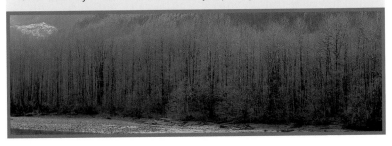

The Squamish River & Salmon

It's hard to tell from up here on the dyke, but if you were to go to the water's edge and stick your hand in, you'd find the water very cold. That's because much of the river's water came from glaciers.

The Squamish River begins about 100 kilometres to the north, among the glaciers of the Pemberton Icefields. Water from melting snow and ice trickles into alpine lakes, forms a river and then runs down, down, downhill. As the Squamish River continues its way south, it is joined by other creeks and rivers such as the Elaho, the Ashlu and the Cheakamus.

The salmon that the eagles feed on at Brackendale hatched either in the Squamish or in its tributaries. When they grew large enough, they swam to the ocean. A few years later, as adults, they returned to the waters where they hatched to lay eggs, thereby starting the whole migration cycle again.

The eagles are part of that cycle. The salmon spawn in gravel beds upstream and then wash down to the lower part of the river, where the eagles rip up the bodies of the dead salmon and eat them. The little bits of salmon that are left over act as fertilizer for algae and other river plants. Insects then eat the algae and the plants. Young salmon eat the insects, thereby completing the food cycle.

There are six species of salmon found in the Squamish River: pink, sockeye, chinook, coho, chum and steelhead. The numbers of some salmon—such as sockeye, chinook, coho and steelhead—are way down from what they used to be. The pink salmon, which was also depleted, is coming back. Because of their numbers—an estimated 150,000 to 450,000 per year—it's the chum salmon that feed the eagles.

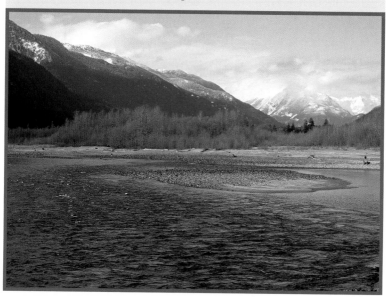

Alice Lake

Length: 4.5-km loop

Time needed: 2 to 2.5 hours

Season: Year-round

Note: The best time to go is spring or autumn; the park is extremely busy in summer.

Rating: Moderate

Dogs: Yes, on leash

Stroller-friendly: All-terrain stroller only

Washrooms: At Alice Lake

Highlights: skunk cabbage, floating gardens, bunchberry, meltwater lakes

Access: Head north on Highway 99 past Squamish and Brackendale and take the turn-off leading eastward to Alice Lake Provincial Park. As you enter the park proper, continue past the campground turn-off and park near the big map and washrooms at Alice Lake.

Driving time: 1.5 hours

Spring is the best time to explore the lakes and trails of Alice Lake Provincial Park, but the park is also a good destination for the short days of winter and the less crowded days of autumn. Come here in summer only if you don't mind crowds.

The hike starts just past the washrooms, across a wooden bridge. Follow the gravel trail right toward the Swamp Lantern Trail. A few minutes later, when you reach a junction, go right again. In another 50 metres there's another junction. This time go left.

The Swamp Lantern Trail loops through a marshy area filled with vine maple, devil's club and skunk cabbage (see p. 112).

Skunk cabbage

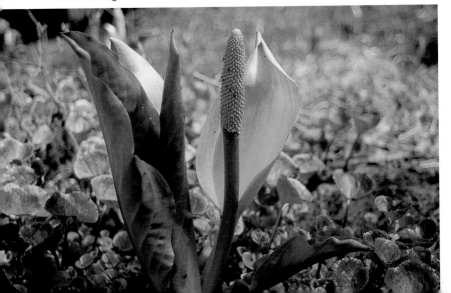

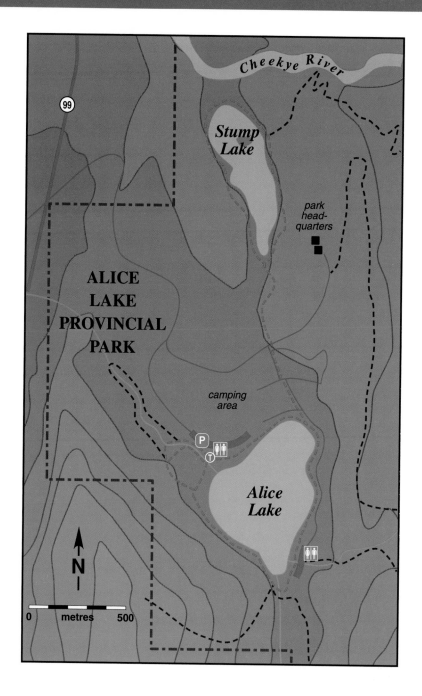

Skunk Cabbage *(Lysichiton americanus)*

Most people call this bright green and yellow plant 'skunk cabbage' because of the way it smells. But there are other names for this plant, such as 'swamp lantern,' which refers to the way that the plant can seem to shine in the darkness of marshes and swamps.

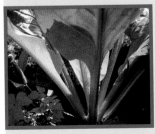

Although we don't use it for much of anything these days, some of BC's First Nations peoples used it for all kinds of things. The large leaves were used to wrap food for storage the way we often use wax paper. The roots were sometimes steamed or roasted and eaten, but only in times of famine.

One Kathlamet First Nation story tells of ancient times before there were ever any salmon and people ate only roots and leaves, including those of the skunk cabbage. When the salmon finally came upriver for the first time, they came ashore and rewarded 'Uncle' Skunk Cabbage for feeding the people. He was given an elk-skin blanket and a war club that he still carries today.

When the loop brings you back to the start, go right and retrace your steps to the first junction. Go right onto the trail that leads to the shores of Alice Lake. (The lake is named after one of the first white people to live in Squamish, Alice Rose, who lived here with her husband, Charles, in the late 1800s.) Follow the lakeside trail through the trees along the western shore. After going up a slight rise, you reach the South Beach.

Stump Lake

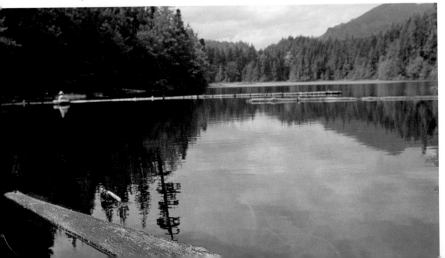

Floating Gardens

In the forest you've probably seen fallen trees called 'nurse logs' that smaller plants and seedlings grow on. But that process doesn't just happen on land; it also happens in the water.

Sometimes when a tree falls into a lake, part of it stays above water. Every now and then a seeds floats by, either on air or on water currents, and lands on that part of the fallen tree. These seeds can sprout here and use the nutrients provided by the decaying tree to grow. After a few years, a fallen tree can look like a floating garden. Depending on what kinds of seeds take root, it can include small plants and shrubs and sometimes even new trees.

Wildlife, especially ducks, love these gardens. Look carefully and you may see ducks resting on top of some of them.

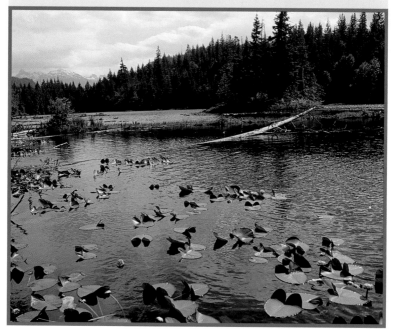

Stay along the lakeshore, following the trail past the picnic tables, then go left and down to cross a wooden bridge over a marshy bit filled with more skunk cabbage. As you continue along the lakeshore, notice how some trees have fallen into the lake. Many of the trees have been there long enough that moss and other plants now grow on them.

Eventually, the trail returns to the North Beach, which is complete with picnic tables and a playground. You might choose to end your hiking day here, or simply pause for lunch.

Bunchberry *(Cornus canadensis)*

Bunchberry in spring or summer has what looks like four-petalled white flowers with a green and purple centre that sticks out. In fact, those white 'petals' are actually bracts, or modified leaves. The actual flowers are the tiny green or purple parts in the middle.

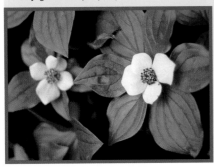

If you see bunchberry in late summer or autumn, when it has a cluster of bright red berries, you'll understand how it got its name—from the bunches of berries that it bears. The berries are sweet but pulpy. Some of BC's coastal First Nations peoples used to eat the berries, both raw and cooked.

To continue to Stump Lake, look for a trail just past the playground that heads toward the parking lot. Follow it across the lot and into the trees, after which it emerges at the campground road. Go right, past campsites 44 to 51, until you reach an information sign. Go left up this road to the main road and cross it. Now you're on the trail to Stump Lake.

As you walk along the trail toward the lake, notice the variety of plants on the forest floor. One of them is bunchberry. Its flower clusters look very similar to the ones that you see on the Pacific dogwood tree—BC's provincial floral emblem and a close relative of bunchberry.

Meltwater Lakes

About 15,000 years ago, a huge glacier covered the Squamish Valley. The ice was so thick that only the tallest mountains—such as Mount Garibaldi, then an active volcano—could be seen on top. The mountains would have looked like little islands in a sea of ice.

But about 12,000 years ago, the climate started to warm again. The ice began to melt and the glacier receded. When that happened, all the lava that had poured out of Garibaldi and turned to rock on the ice sheet tumbled down the mountain slopes.

Soon, the melting water from the glacier began to trickle through all the rock and rubble, carving out a channel. Eventually, the amount of water trickling through slowed. And finally all that was left behind were some of the deeper places filled with water—Alice Lake and Stump Lake.

Not much farther along the trail, you come to the south end of Stump Lake. Go right and follow the trail around the east side of the lake, past clusters of pond-lilies, buckbean and hardhack. You also pass a little island, covered in trees. It is the big version of the floating gardens that you saw at Alice Lake.

Eventually the trail comes to the north end of Stump Lake. Follow the trail sign that points you straight ahead to continue the Stump Lake Loop. About 5 to 10 minutes along the loop trail, watch on the left for an old cedar tree that has fallen and become a side trail to a marsh. There you can see cattails, buckbean and, if you're lucky, in spring you may see tadpoles.

The loop trail then passes through a darker, denser forest than on the other side of the lake. Notice how the trees are all pretty skinny? And how there are stumps scattered throughout the forest? The reason is that you are in a fairly young second-growth forest. The big trees were cut down more than 70 years ago. It'll take centuries before this area is covered in old-growth forest again.

The trail climbs to a viewpoint. If there are no clouds, look for part of Mount Garibaldi in the distance. An information sign here tells you some of the geological history of this area, including how Alice and Stump lakes came to be.

The trail drops back down and returns you to the south end of Stump Lake. Now all you need to do is retrace your steps to the main road, through the campground and back to the parking lot at Alice Lake.

Mount Garibaldi in cloud

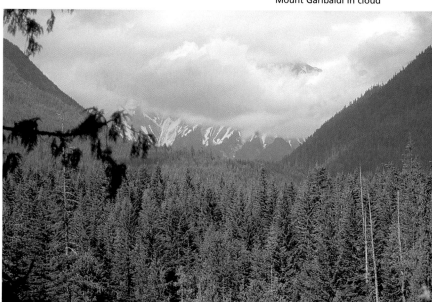

Brandywine Falls

Length: 4.5 km

Time needed: 2 to 2.5 hours

Season: May to October

Rating: Easy

Dogs: Yes, on leash

Stroller-friendly: All-terrain stroller only

Washrooms: At Brandywine Provincial Park

Highlights: Lodgepole pine, basalt columns, lava lakes, falls

Access: From Horseshoe Bay, take Highway 99 northward past Squamish. After the Daisy Lake Reservoir, watch for the blue and white Brandywine Provincial Park signs. The park is on the right, just after a railway crossing.

Driving time: 2 hours

Brandywine Falls, the highlight of Brandywine Park, is visited by thousands of people each year. Few people, however, hike the trails here and see the other treasures—including evidence of ancient volcanoes and glaciers—tucked among the trees.

From the day-use area at Brandywine Provincial Park, head toward the sound of Brandywine Creek. Cross the bridge and go left. The first 100 metres or so is steep, but it's the only uphill that you'll do on this hike. Soon enough, the trail levels and you pass under a powerline.

As you go up a slight hill on the right, there's a small marshy area that often has odd-looking little mushrooms growing among the sedges. Also notice the trees around you. There's one species in particular growing here that you won't see in the rainforests around Vancouver: the lodgepole pine (although you may see its close relative, the shore pine, here and there).

Lodgepole Pine *(Pinus contorta* var. *latifolia)*

The easiest way to identify lodgepole pine is by its needles, which come in bundles of two. It has cones that look like miniature pineapples.

The lodgepole pine grows easily in places where forest fires have burned. Although fire might kill many lodgepole pine trees, it is also an important factor in the growth of new ones. The heat of the fire melts the resin in the lodge-

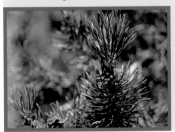

pole pine's cones, releasing the seeds and allowing them to fall to the scorched forest floor, where they can sprout and grow.

The lodgepole pine got its name from the explorers Lewis and Clark, who noticed that First Nations people used poles from this tall, straight tree to support teepees and lodges.

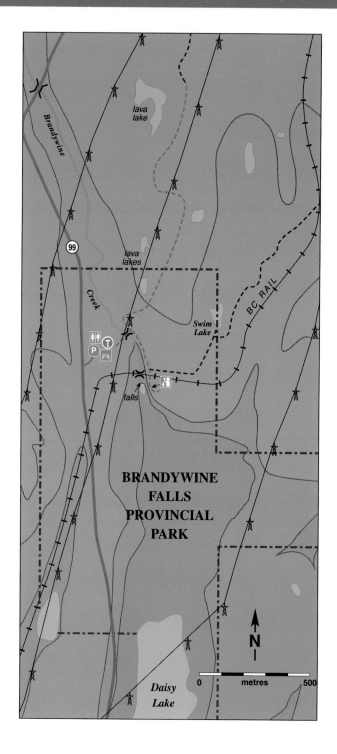

lava
lake

Brandywine

99

lava
lakes

Creek

Swim
Lake

B.C. RAIL

falls

BRANDYWINE
FALLS
PROVINCIAL
PARK

N

0   metres   500

Daisy
Lake

As you continue along the trail, notice the many different tree and plant species.

Also be sure to check out the trail itself. From time to time the dirt gives way to what looks like interlocking patio bricks. But they are not bricks—they are rock that was created a long time ago by a volcano and a glacier.

Basalt Columns

It's believed that somewhere between 11,000 and 15,000 years ago, Mount Garibaldi erupted. The lava that flowed out was made of basalt, a dark-coloured rock that is rich in magnesium and iron.

When basaltic lava cools, it shrinks. Sometimes when it shrinks it cracks in a particular hexagonal (six-sided, like a honeycomb) pattern. This process 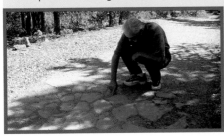 is called 'columnar jointing.' It starts on the surface of the lava and gradually creeps farther inward as the molten rock inside also cools. What you're seeing beneath your feet is the tops of some of those columns.

Lava Lakes

These little lakes are called 'lava lakes' not because they were formed by lava, but because they lie in rock that once was lava.

If you walk around the lake, you can see the same 'tiles' of basaltic columns as you saw on the trail. Over time, small depressions formed in the rock when 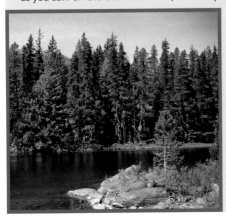 parts of it settled and other parts were lifted up by geologic forces. Water trickled in and filled the depressions.

With a constant water source, various species of plants were able to grow and now things look quite lush and green along the lakeshore. In some cases, though, the plants will eventually take over until the lake becomes completely overgrown and disappears.

The trail leads on over more of the patterned rock and past more tiny lakelets until soon you come to a part of the trail that lies between two bigger lakes. (Sometimes rainfall puts the trail under a bit of water and these two lakes become one.) In late spring you can see typical marsh plants (such as bog-laurel, buckthorn and Labrador tea) in bloom here. Follow the trail for another 10 minutes or so until you find another lava lake.

Turn around and retrace your steps to the bridge where you started. Don't cross it just yet. Instead, go straight ahead to see Brandywine Falls. You will need to cross some railway tracks. Be careful to listen for the sound of a train coming.

At the junction just on the other side, go right, and, in 5 to 10 minutes, you will come to a viewpoint that overlooks Brandywine Falls.

When you're finished soaking in the views, retrace your steps over the bridge and back to the parking lot.

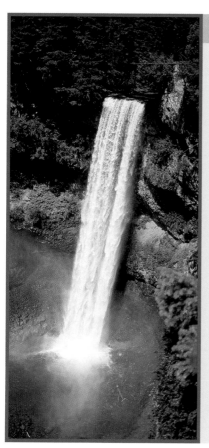

Brandywine Falls

The waters of Brandywine Creek drop 66 metres before continuing. Look across at the cliffs on the other side and you may notice that the rock is made of layers, each with a slightly different colour to it. Each of those layers represents a different lava flow. For thousands of years, before any people lived here, Mount Garibaldi was a volcano that erupted every few thousand years. During each eruption it spewed out molten lava that worked its way from the volcano down into the valley here.

A few thousand years ago, Brandywine Falls fell close to where you're standing today. But the water is continually eroding the rock underneath and the falls continues to move back, bit by tiny bit, each year. If you were to come back in another few thousand years, you might find the falls somewhere close to where you parked your car.

Rainbow Falls

Length: 5 km

Time needed: 2.5 to 3 hours

Season: May to October

Rating: Tough; elevation gain of 150 metres—best for ages eight and older

Dogs: Yes, on leash

Stroller-friendly: No

Washrooms: Outhouse near turn-around point

Highlights: Waterfall, big boulders, old forest fire, mountain views

Note: Keep a close eye on kids and don't let them too near the falls. The rocks can be slippery.

Access: Follow Highway 99 northward to Whistler. After crossing the railway tracks and Function Junction (at Alpha Lake Road), turn left onto Alta Lake Road and continue for about 7 kilometres. Just after the sign for Rainbow Park on the right there is a sign for the Rainbow Lake Trail on the left. Park here, at the mouth of Twentyone Mile Creek.

Driving time: 2 hours

Hikers have been visiting Rainbow Falls since the early 1900s, long before the resort municipality of Whistler came into being. It's easy to understand why. The falls themselves are gorgeous and the forest provides lots to see. It's also a good hike to do on a hot day because both the shade of the forest and the spray of the falls will help keep you cool.

The trail starts on the south side of the creek (the left side if you're looking upstream). Follow it up through the trees for about 200 metres to where the trail forks. Bear right, staying along the creek.

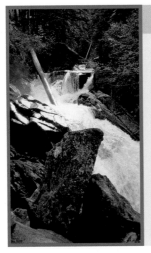

Rainbow Falls

Notice how some of the rocks here are smooth and rounded? Almost as if someone had rubbed them with a giant piece of sandpaper? Well, in a way, that's what happened, only it was the effect of the water—and the pebbles and grit that it carries—pounding away on the rock surface over thousands of years.

A waterfall is one place where you can easily see the power of water. (It's harder to see in a wide river because that power is spread over a large area.) Because the creek is so powerful here, it can be dangerous: stay far away from the edge.

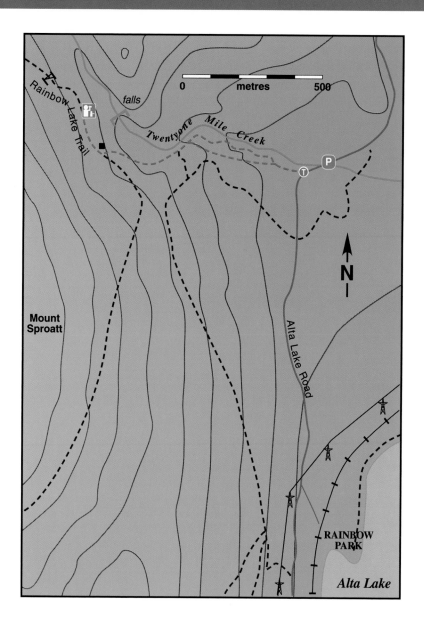

In another few minutes there's another junction. Go right, following the sign for Rainbow Falls. The trail is steep, so take your time and stop to check out the flowers and shrubs along the way. About 15 minutes later you will arrive at another junction. Follow the trail downward and under a fallen tree to the falls. If the light hits the mist just right, you might even see a rainbow.

Big Boulders

Some of these boulders are as big as cars, some even as big as houses. But notice how they aren't smooth like the other rocks that you saw just upstream? That difference can mean one of two things: they could be made of a different, harder kind of rock than the others, or they might have been

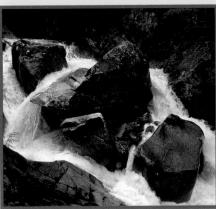

in the creek for a lot less time.

In this case, the big boulders are a more recent addition to the creek. It's likely that they were part of a big rockfall that came from the steep slope across the creek and that they rolled downhill until they landed in the creek. If you were to come back here hundreds of years from now, you'd find smaller, smoother boulders than you see today.

Forest Fire

In 1951, a logging company decided to log this side of the creek. People who lived nearby and people who hiked here asked them not to cut the old-growth trees, but the company went ahead and did so.

After logging part of the mountain, the company set fire to the slash (all the branches, scraps and smaller trees for which they had no use). But the fire got out of control and burned for three weeks, moving into the still-standing forest and all the way to the bluffs of Mount Sproatt high above.

Fire can cause some important—and beneficial—changes in a forest ecosystem. Certain tree species, such as lodgepole pine, need fire to melt the resin in their cones and release the seeds within. And certain shrubs, such as ceanothus (also known as buckbrush because it's a favourite food of deer and elk) need fire to prepare the seed for sprouting.

Fire can also create openings in the forest that let other plants and trees grow. And it helps recycle many of the nutrients contained in burned trees and other plants (including slash): the ash resulting from the fire is dissolved by rain and melting snow and returned to the soil where it can be used by other plants.

Unfortunately, in this case, because of the amount of forest burned, the fire did more harm than good. The trees are growing back now, but the forest will take a very long time to recover.

Follow the trail a little farther downslope for another view of the waterfall. In the middle of the creek lie a number of huge boulders (see p. 122).

Go back to the last junction and turn right in the direction indicated by the Rainbow Lake sign. A short, steep hike will bring you to a gravel road right next to a water supply building.

Continue up the road past the sign that indicates that there is an outhouse ahead. You will soon see the part of Rainbow Creek above the falls and even the top of the falls themselves. Because Whistler's drinking water comes from this creek, the area has been fenced off.

About 10 to 15 minutes later on the road is the outhouse. Keep going along the road a bit farther. Look at the forest on this side of Rainbow Creek and the forest on the other side of the creek. Notice the difference?

On this side of the creek there are small, young trees and lots of tall, bare snags—the trunks of dead trees that look like flagpoles without the flag. But across the creek it's greener, with older, taller trees that have lichen hanging from their branches. Why the difference? The clue is in the blackened stumps that you can see on the slope above you.

Continue up the road for five minutes or so, to a viewpoint (see below).

The trail ahead continues for another 5.5 kilometres to Rainbow Lake— best saved for a day when you've got lots of energy and lots of time. Otherwise, just turn around and retrace your steps back to the parking area.

Mountain Views

From the viewpoint, you can see Whistler Valley and the mountains on the other side. Green Lake is on the left, with Wedge Mountain, Parkhurst Mountain and Weart Mountain towering above. You can also see Blackcomb and Whistler mountains with their criss-crosses of ski runs. Much of Blackcomb was logged in the 1940s. The trees were hauled down to a mill that used to be at Lost Lake. Whistler Mountain was logged in the mid-1960s as part of its transformation to a ski resort.

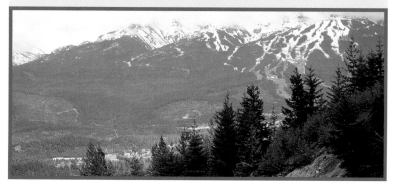

Lost Lake

Length: 5-km loop
Time needed: 2 to 2.5 hours
Season: May to October
Rating: Easy
Dogs: Yes, on leash
Stroller-friendly: All-terrain stroller only
Washrooms: Outhouses at Lost Lake

Highlights: Glacial creeks, western white pine, marsh, beach
Access: Follow Highway 99 north to Whistler Village. Turn right at Village Gate Boulevard and follow it to a T junction. Turn left on Blackcomb Way and follow the signs to the parking lot for the Lost Lake trails.
Driving time: 2 hours

Lost Lake is a popular stop for families looking for a warm, shallow place to swim on a hot summer Whistler day. Although the beach may be packed with people, the trails are not; they are also wide and offer lots to see, from wildflowers to mountain views.

From the parking lot, head toward the sound of rushing water, Fitzsimmons Creek. A wide gravel path leads under an overpass and then over a wooden bridge. Stop and take a look upstream where a side creek joins Fitzsimmons (see below).

Cross the bridge. On the other side there is a map of the Lost Lake trails. Follow the main trail up about 200 metres and keep right at the next two junctions to stay on the main trail. At the third junction, keep right again and follow the green Lost Lake Loop signs.

Along the way, take note of the trees that grow alongside the trail. There's one kind of pine tree here that you don't see very often (see p. 126).

Creek Origins

The most noticeable difference between Fitzsimmons Creek and Blackcomb Creek is colour. Fitzsimmons varies from light green to light blue, but Blackcomb is darker and can be blue, or sometimes brownish.

The different colours result from the different places where each creek begins. Fitzsimmons Creek starts high in the mountains, where Fitzsimmons Glacier is melted by sun and rain. Glaciers have a lot of fine, ground-up rock (rock flour) in them that gets carried away in the meltwater.

Blackcomb Creek flows out of Lost Lake, where there are no glaciers but there are lots of trees, shrubs and other vegetation. It's when there's a lot of dead vegetation (such as fallen autumn leaves) in the lake that the creek water can look a little brownish.

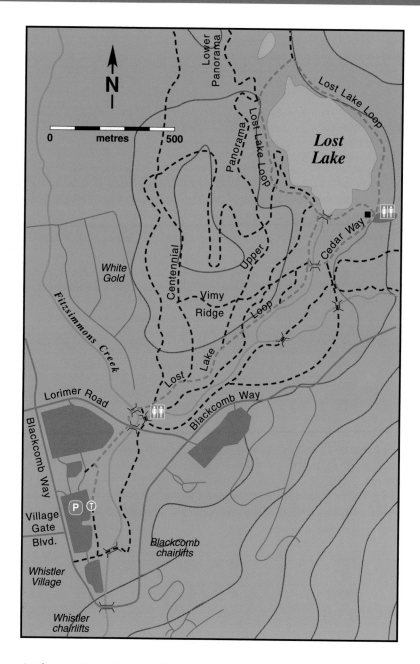

At the next junction, go right to follow the Cedar Way Trail. You first cross a bridge over Blackcomb Creek. About 25 metres farther, the gravel road gives way to pavement. Stay left and cross a bridge over Horstmann Creek. A little farther, another bridge will take you across Blackcomb Creek again.

Western White Pine *(Pinus monticola)*

In southwestern BC, there are three species of native pine—shore pine and lodgepole pine (varieties of *Pinus contorta*), whitebark pine (*Pinus albicaulis*) and western white pine. You can tell two of them apart by the number of needles in a bundle: shore pine has two needles, but western white pine has five; whitebark pine also has five, but it is found only at much higher elevations.

The other way to recognize a western white pine is by its cones, which are long and skinny, about the size of a banana. In contrast, shore pine cones are short and stubby and about the size of a small chicken egg.

Pinus contorta is now more common than western white pine, but it was not always that way. A fungus called white pine blister rust came to Vancouver in 1910 on some eastern white pine trees imported from France. Within 12 years 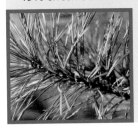 the fungus had spread everywhere the native western white pines grew, killing many young trees.

Some western white pines seem to have a natural resistance to the fungus. Scientists are trying to figure out how the resistance works, so they can breed new western white pines that won't fall victim to the disease.

Stay straight ahead on the paved path past the warming hut used by cross-country skiers in winter, and you will arrive at the eastern end of Lost Lake. There are washrooms and picnic tables here.

After visiting East Beach, return to the same path and continue northward along the gravel section. In summer, lupine, Indian paintbrush and other wildflowers grow along the trail. A bit farther along is a big floating dock. You can scramble down the slope to check it out.

Return to the main trail and continue north to reach the next junction, where there are signs and a map.

Lost Lake

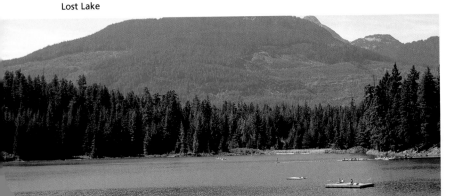

The Value of Marshes

Although a beach can be nice for people, it's not always a good thing for animals. That's because marshes provide food and shelter in ways that a beach can't. Marshes provide plant materials that some insects like to feed on and lay eggs on. Those insects might then become food for other insects or for frogs, toads, turtles, fish and salamanders.

Those insect-eating animals also need the marsh plants and watery environment for shelter, for breeding and to help hide them from other animals that feed on them. Some of the mammals that hang around marshes include shrews, muskrats, beavers, otters and coyotes.

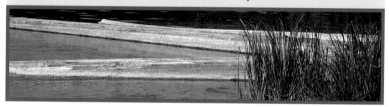

Go left and take the Lost Lake Loop Trail to head back along the other side of the lake. (You could make up a longer loop, using trails such as the Old Mill Road and Lower and Upper Panorama).

Not much farther along you will reach the west end of Lost Lake, where there is a small marsh. Before sand was brought in to make East Beach suitable for swimming, it looked much like this end of the lake.

Continue along the trail to the next junction and keep left. You'll arrive back at the east end of the lake. To the left you'll see more of the remaining marsh. There is also a footbridge that crosses two creeks.

Return to the junction and continue straight ahead on the trail that will rejoin the main trail. Or continue to the beach area again and return the way you came, back to the parking lot.

Inlet & Outlet Creeks

The water necessary to fill up a lake and keep it full has to come from somewhere. Although rain and snow do contribute directly, most of the water comes from 'inlet creeks' that flow into the lake. When a new lake forms, the water can get only so high before it overflows somewhere. An 'outlet creek' develops at the place where the water overflows.

If the lake lies at a low point between some hills or mountain peaks, the inlet creeks usually enter where the land is higher. The outlet creek is where there is the biggest gap between the hills or peaks. In the case of Lost Lake, however, both the inlet and outlet creeks are found at the same end.

Cougar Mountain

Length: 6 km

Time needed: 2.5 to 3 hours

Season: May to October

Rating: Moderate; elevation gain of 150 metres, some rough trail—best for ages eight and up

Dogs: Yes, on leash

Stroller-friendly: No

Washrooms: None

Highlights: Lichen, old-growth forests, western redcedar, devil's club

Access: From Whistler Village, take Highway 99 north for 9 kilometres. Just past Green Lake, on the west side of the highway, is the Sixteen Mile Creek Forest Service Road. Turn left across the highway and onto the road. Stay right at the first fork. At the next fork, 4 kilometres farther, stay right again. An additional 1 kilometre brings you to a third fork. If you've got a two-wheel-drive vehicle, park here. If you're four-wheeling, you can continue for another 0.7 kilometres up a rather rough road.

Driving time: (from Whistler Village) 20 minutes

Follow the road as it climbs gradually, being sure to watch for 4 x 4 vehicles and mountain bikes coming both up and down. You will come to the first steep and rocky bit (about 50 metres or so). Then the road levels briefly before resuming its rocky climb.

Take a break at the first hairpin turn and look down into the tiny valley scattered with little water-lilied ponds. Not much farther is the start of the trail proper. The first sign that you're about to enter an older forest is that the trees are suddenly taller and bigger than any you've seen so far on the hike. The second sign is the light green lichen that hangs from the trees here (see p. 130).

Showh Lakes viewpoint

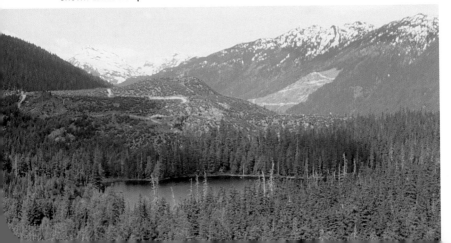

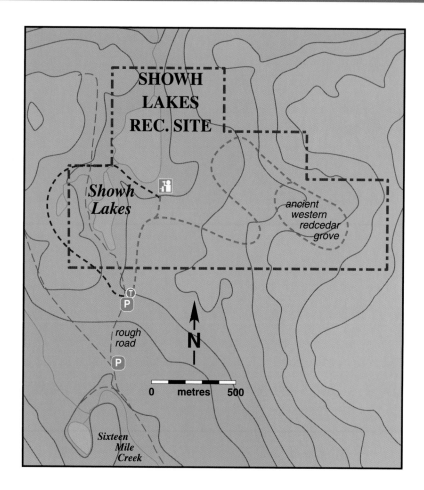

Follow the trail up and over a rock outcrop and then down again. You will pass a plank bench. A bit farther, just about where you start to hear a stream up ahead, look for a side trail on the left that leads to a viewpoint.

From here you can see the Showh Lakes below, and, in the distance, three mountains: Sisqa, Semam and Kwtamts. Also take a few minutes to compare old-growth and second-growth forests (see p. 130).

Retrace your steps to the main trail and follow it to a wooden bridge and across a tiny creek. Just past where a big Douglas-fir recently crashed down on the trail, the big trees begin. The biggest of them all are the western redcedars that Cougar Mountain is known for (see p. 131).

The trail continues past big trees and over a couple of small wooden bridges as it loops around. In the warmer seasons, you may notice that there are mosquitoes and other bugs around. They're here for the same reason that the western redcedars are—because it's damp. There are also other moisture-loving plants that live here, such as skunk cabbage and devil's club (see p. 131).

Eventually the creek trail loops around until you come back to the creek and the very first bridge that you crossed over. Just go left and retrace your steps back down the trail and logging road.

Common Witch's Hair Lichen
(Alectoria sarmentosa)

There are more than 1000 different species of lichen in our part of the world. Some of them are very rare, but you can often see common witch's hair in mountain forests.

This lichen was used by First Nations people in bandages, diapers, clothing and footwear, and as hair for decorating dance masks.

Common witch's hair lichen is also an important winter food for wildlife, including deer, caribou, mountain goats and moose. This lichen is also used for building nests by small mammals such as voles and chipmunks and by birds such as hawks and hummingbirds.

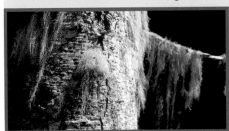

Lichens take a very long time to grow. Though some grow slower than others, most lichens grow only about one millimetre (the width of a pencil-lead) each year. Some of them can be as much as 4000 years old.

Old-growth & Second-growth Forests

First look on the mountain slope to your left for the big brown patch of a recent clearcut. Directly in front are some areas that were clearcut 5 to 15 years ago. A second-growth forest has begun to grow there.

Finally, there's the forest that you're sitting in: old-growth. As you can imagine, more kinds of plants and animals tend to live in old-growth forests than in clearcuts or even in second-growth forests, just because there tends to be more food, shelter and diversity in old-growth than the others.

Some plants and animals do live quite happily in second-growth forests. But many people—including scientists—believe that it's important to have both old-growth and second-growth forests. And since it would take a very, very long time for replanted forests to become old-growth, we need to make sure that we save the old-growth that we have left.

Devil's Club *(Oplopanax horridus)*

The first thing to know about devil's club is that it is a plant that you don't want to touch. Both the leaves and the stem have sharp, pointy spikes that hurt even if you just brush against them. (The spikes also break off easily and can stay in your skin and become infected.)

Despite its nastiness, devil's club is still an important part of the forest. Bears eat the red berries that come out in autumn. (People, however, should not eat them, because they are considered inedible.) And BC's First Nations peoples used the plant for everything from fishing lures to dyes to medicines for such ailments as arthritis, tuberculosis and measles.

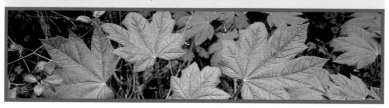

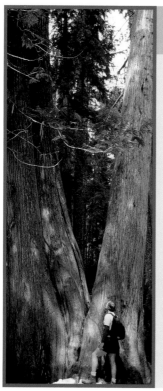

Western Redcedar
(Thuja plicata)

Some of the trees on Cougar Mountain are more than 60 metres tall (taller than 30 adult men standing one on top of the other) and almost 10 metres around (it would take 5 or more men standing fingertip to fingertip to wrap their arms around the biggest tree).

These trees are also very old—from 600 to 1000 years old. When the oldest tree here was just a little seedling, Vikings were raiding the British Isles and the Maori people were settling in New Zealand.

The western redcedar is the provincial tree of BC. It has been used by many of BC's native peoples for hundreds of years. They made clothing from the bark and baskets from the roots. They used its wood for tools, houses, canoes, totem poles and much more. To see some of the ways that redcedar has been used, visit the Vancouver Museum or the University of British Columbia's Museum of Anthropology.

Iona Beach

Length: 4 km

Time needed: 2 to 2.5 hours

Season: Year-round

Rating: Easy

Dogs: No

Stroller-friendly: No

Washrooms: At parking lot

Highlights: Beach pea, yellow-headed blackbirds, large-headed sedge, beach hoppers

Access: Head southward over the Oak Street Bridge to Richmond. Take the first exit and follow the signs for Vancouver International Airport westward along Sea Island Way. Cross the Moray Swing Bridge, then take the first right, and then, immediately afterward, another right onto Grauer Road. Follow the Iona Beach Regional Park signs for about another 12 kilometres, past the Iona Sewage Treatment Plant, to the parking area.

Driving time: 30 minutes

From the parking lot, head to the boardwalk for the south pond. No matter what time of year, you'll see a good variety of ducks and other waterfowl here. In spring and summer, for example, there are three kinds of teal: cinnamon, blue-winged and green-winged. In autumn and winter there are northern pintail ducks and northern shovelers.

Walk northward on the boardwalk and back to the shore and continue north along the sandy path. If you're here in late spring or summer, take a moment to look for a pretty little plant with pink-purple flowers.

Beach Pea *(Lathyrus japonicus)*

This plant might look similar to one of the plants in your garden at home, the sweet pea. That's because they're in the same family—Fabaceae (Leguminosae). The difference is that beach pea is a wild plant that is native to BC and sweet pea is a cultivated plant that is not native to BC.

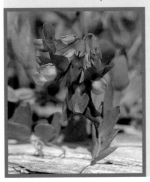

If you look closely at beach pea, you can see pea pods that look just like the ones you sometimes eat at home. In fact, native peoples of BC ate beach peas raw or boiled or preserved in seal oil. When the pea pods are ripe, they turn black; for that reason the Haida people called this plant 'Raven's Canoe.'

Although this particular species of pea is edible, other species that look similar are not—in fact, they can be poisonous. So, it's best to just look and touch, but not eat, this pea.

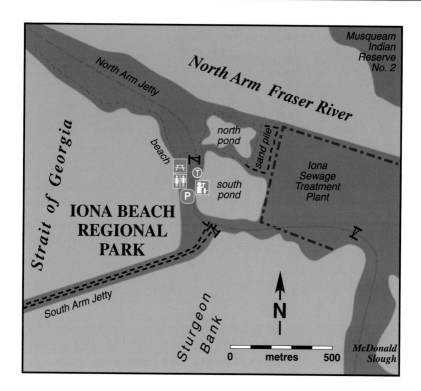

When you come to a point between the two ponds, go right along a path lined with broom, wild roses and other plants. You're going to be walking around the north pond, but, as you do, be sure to keep your eyes and ears open for yellow-headed blackbirds.

Iona ponds

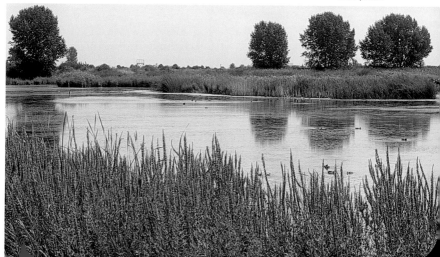

Yellow-headed Blackbird
(Xanthocephalus xanthocephalus)

The yellow-headed blackbird is a bit bigger than its close relative the red-winged blackbird (see p. 26). The male looks as if he's wearing a bright yellow hood. The female is a little smaller and is brown with yellow on her throat and breast. Even if you don't see any of these birds right away, you'll likely hear the loud *krraaaak* that is their call.

Yellow-headed blackbirds eat insects and seeds. They build their nests up high above the water, often attached to a cattail.

Unlike the red-winged blackbird, which can be seen all over the Lower Mainland, Iona Beach is the best of only a few places to see the yellow-headed blackbird.

Be sure to go left and follow the path that curves around the north pond heading toward the North Arm of the Fraser River, then left again so that you're on a pathway between the pond and the river. Take a moment to watch the boat traffic on the river. You'll see fishing boats, barges and maybe even a canoe or two. Occasionally, you might even see a harbour seal swimming by.

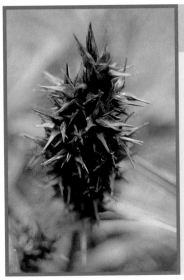

Large-headed Sedge
(Carex macrocephala)

One very noticeable plant growing here is the large-headed sedge. It has a skinny stem with, just as the name suggests, a big head of sharp, brown spikes. These spikes are the plant's flowers.

This sedge has male flowers on one plant and female flowers on another. Wind takes pollen from male to female flowers, and the female flowers form the seeds. Sometimes animals—including people—help spread the seeds when the seed's covering catches in fur, feathers or a sock or shoe.

Follow the path back to a gravel road and go across. You're now wandering over the sand dunes toward the sea, but watch where you walk. Otherwise you might step on some of the spikier plants that live here.

Once you're past the sand dunes, you'll hit the beach. Head northwest along the North Arm Jetty for about 30 minutes. You'll see lots of interesting stuff, including driftwood, shells and beach hoppers.

If the tide is low, you can head back along the mud-flats, checking out the birds, the clams and other marine life seen here. You will return to the parking area where you started.

Beach Hoppers (Family Orchestidae)

If you sit on the beach for even a little while, you'll probably notice some beach hoppers. They're also called sand fleas, but, despite that name, they're not fleas. In fact, they're not even insects. Beach hoppers are crustaceans, so they're actually related to shrimps, crabs and lobsters.

Beach hoppers are very small—about the same size as a child's pinky fingernail. They look like very teeny tiny shrimp and have seven body segments with five pairs of long legs that they use for swimming and jumping. They hop around in sand and on driftwood and especially around seaweed as they look for dead and decaying seaweed or animals to eat.

During the day, beach hoppers spend most of their time staying moist by burrowing into the sand or into seaweed. As night falls, they come out and hop all over the beach in their search for supper. To hop, beach hoppers bend their bodies double and then let go with a jerk, springing forward using a tail-like appendage. They've been known to jump up to 50 centimetres—about 100 times their own body length—in a single leap.

Iona Beach

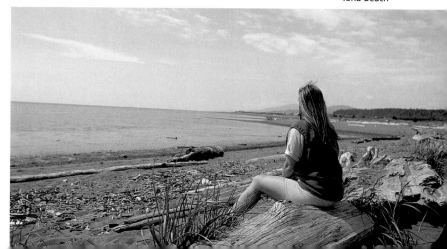

Richmond Nature Park

Length: 5.5-km loop

Time needed: 2 to 2.5 hours

Season: Year-round

Note: Most bog plants are in flower during May and June.

Rating: Easy

Dogs: Not allowed

Stroller-friendly: All-terrain stroller only

Washrooms: Inside the Nature House

Highlights: Blueberries, Labrador tea, bog, spotted towhee

Access: Take Highway 99 south to exit 38 (Shell Road, Richmond Centre). Follow Shell Road south, past the stoplight at Alderbridge Way, to Westminster Highway and turn left. Watch for the signs pointing to the park and turn left into the parking area.

Driving time: 25 minutes

Deep in the heart of Richmond lies a 40-hectare hidden treasure. You may have even passed by in a car or bus and never known it was there. But, tucked behind the trees, there is an unusual bog park, with walking paths lined with blueberry bushes and evergreen trees, as well as plants usually seen only in places much farther north.

Blueberries & Birds

Although the berries may all be blue and look pretty much the same at first glance, there are in fact lots of different species of blueberries (*Vaccinium* spp.) growing in Richmond Nature Park. Some of them are native to the Lower Mainland, but most of them are varieties that were brought to the area from other places and planted by farmers.

The most interesting thing about the blueberry bushes that you see here is that they weren't planted by people, but by birds. How? Imagine a bird eating blueberries at a nearby blueberry farm. A little while later it flies over the park and poops. The blueberry seeds in the bird poop (which have passed through the bird undigested) land on fertile ground and sprout, and a new blueberry bush grows.

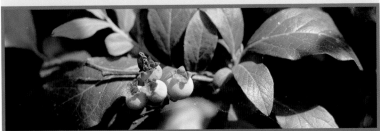

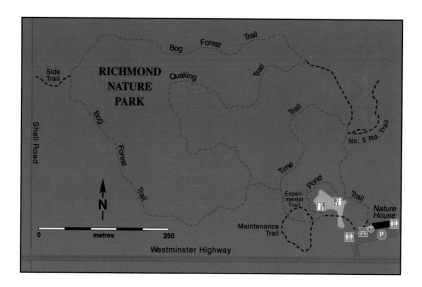

Make your first stop the Nature House. Here you can pick up a trail guide and other information about the park. (Save the gift-shop browse for your return.) Once back outside, follow the boardwalk behind the Nature House. About 50 metres along on the left there is a platform with a bench. You can see part of the duck pond from here. Not much farther there is a junction.

Go right and walk along a bark mulch path lined with salal, Labrador tea and blueberry bushes.

Labrador Tea *(Ledum groenlandicum)*

Pick a leaf off the Labrador tea bush. (The leaf should be green on top, and brown and slightly fuzzy underneath. If it isn't, then it isn't Labrador tea.) Crush the leaf in your hand and then sniff it—it smells great.

Some people make tea using these leaves. They pick them, wash them and pour boiling water over them. After a few minutes, the water takes on the taste and the scent of the leaves.

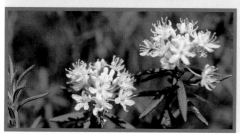

Warning: It's important to be sure that the leaves are those of Labrador tea. Similar leaves of other bog plants, such as bog-laurel, bog-rosemary and trapper's tea, are thought to contain toxic substances.

Understanding Bogs

To understand what a bog is, it's important to understand how a bog is formed. It all started a very long time ago—about 10,000 years ago—when huge ice sheets melted away. The land that had been squashed under the weight of all the ice began to rise—although it was still underwater. Then, over the next few thousand years, the Fraser River carried down sand, clay and other kinds of very fine dirt and deposited it here. Soon, the land was above water. Plants began to grow. And when they died, they formed layer upon layer of stuff called peat.

Then a certain type of moss, called sphagnum, began to grow. It can absorb a lot of water, like a sponge. That's what makes the ground so springy.

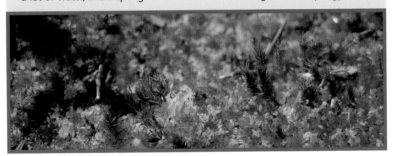

After about 10 minutes of walking you reach another junction. Go left to follow the Time Trail, which takes you toward the heart of the bog. You'll see more plants, such as Labrador tea, shore pine and other types of plants that can live in these boggy conditions.

At the next trail junction, go right. Another 25 metres farther there is another junction. Go right again to follow the Quaking Trail. About 10 to 15 minutes later you'll come to a bench. Take a moment to sit down. In May or June, take a closer look at the little white flowers all around. They belong to the Labrador tea.

As you continue your walk, notice how in some places the trail seems wetter and squishier. If you jump up and down, the ground feels springy, not hard like regular ground, and a puddle of water will appear. That's because the ground you're walking on is bog.

Continue to the next junction. For a short outing of about 4 kilometres (instead of the full 5.5-kilometre loop), you can go right here and return to the Nature House. But, if you're still up for more, have a snack break and then go left on the Bog Forest Trail. Here you can walk under the branches of western white birch, western hemlock and other trees that live on the edges of the bog. This part of the park is also a good place to see the spotted towhee.

Spotted Towhee *(Pipilo maculatus)*

Bigger than a sparrow, but smaller than a robin, the spotted towhee (formerly known as the rufous-sided towhee) looks as if it's wearing a black coat with a black hood. It has small, ruby red eyes and splashes of rusty red feathers on its sides. Its belly is white and there are also white spots on its back and wings.

One of the best places to find a spotted towhee is on the ground, where towhees look for food. You can usually hear them scratching away among the dead leaves beneath trees and shrubs as these birds look for seeds, bugs and berries and sometimes even snakes.

The bird's name comes from the call that it makes: *toe-whee.*

After walking for 30 to 40 minutes from the last junction, you come to a junction that you passed earlier. Go right, and, 25 metres farther, go right again. At the next junction, go left, following the sign for the Nature House. Then, almost immediately, go left again. This trail connects with the main trail. Go left once more and follow the trail to the pond.

To walk around the pond (a five-minute trip), go left on the boardwalk. Hidden among all the pond plants there are some turtles and frogs. These species are not native to this park or to BC; they were brought here by people who owned them as pets. Then just follow the signs back to the Nature House and the parking lot.

For information on the Nature Park's hours, call (604) 718-6188.

Richmond Nature Park

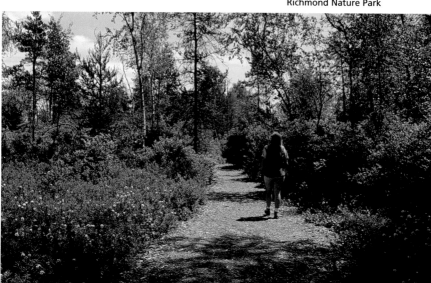

Deas Island

Length: 4.5-km loop

Time needed: 2 to 2.5 hours

Season: Year-round

Rating: Easy

Dogs: Yes, on leash

Stroller-friendly: Yes, except for 200 m of Sand Dune Trail (accessible with all-terrain stroller)

Washrooms: Outhouses at Riverside and Fisher's Field picnic areas

Highlights: Old cannery relics, cottonwood trees, horsetails, Cooper's hawks

Access: Follow Highway 99 south to Ladner and take exit 28 (the Tsawwassen and Ferries exit). Stay in the leftmost of the two exit lanes and follow the signs for River Road left over the overpass and onto 62B Street. About 2.3 kilometres farther, turn at the left-turn lane for Deas Island Regional Park and drive to the Riverside picnic area.

Driving time: 45 minutes

Tucked just off Highway 99 amidst a mix of farmland and industrial parks is a breath of fresh air: 70-hectare Deas Island. Here you'll find trails that follow the Fraser River and wander in and out of sun-dappled forest that opens in places to give views of the river.

From the picnic area, follow the path along the river. On a clear day there are great views of the mountains surrounding the Lower Mainland, all the way from the peaks of the Tetrahedron on the Sunshine Coast to the summits in Golden Ears Provincial Park.

You soon arrive at a cairn that notes some of Deas Island's history. Go right and along the boardwalk to the viewing tower. From the top you can see way down the Fraser River's South Arm.

Once you're down from the tower, head back toward the information signboard and go right, past an old boiler, to the Tinmaker's Walk. That name refers to a man who used to live on the island (see p. 141).

Tinmaker's Walk

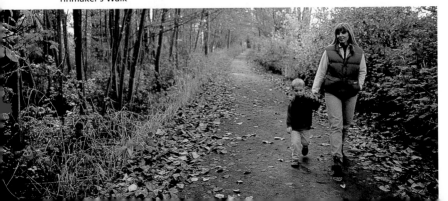

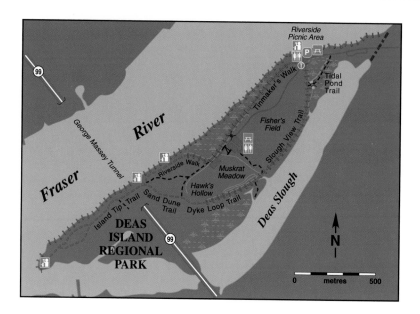

The Old Cannery

John Sullivan Deas was a freed slave who had come to Canada from South Carolina with his wife and eight children. He came to this island and set up a tin can–making operation for a small salmon canning company that was nearby.

When the owner of that cannery died, Deas decided to can salmon himself. So, in 1873, he built dykes to keep the river from flooding some of the land, then built cannery buildings and a wharf. For three years, his cannery produced more cases of tinned salmon per year than any other cannery on the Fraser River.

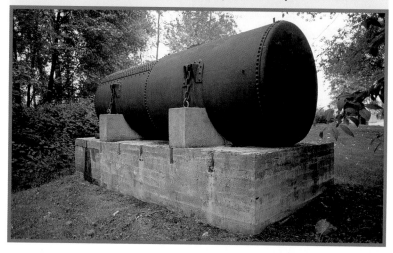

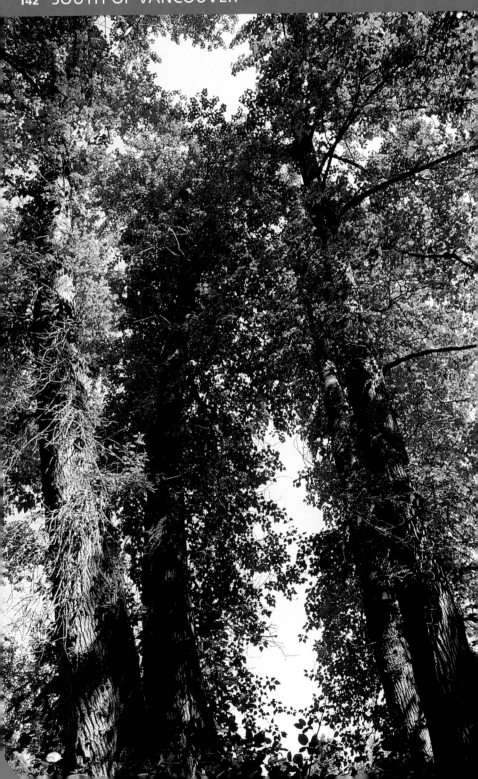

The trail is lined with alder and cottonwood trees and many kinds of shrubs that provide food and shelter for songbirds. This part of the park is what Deas Island most likely looked like years and years ago, before people came to the island. In those days it was just one of many sandbar islands created by the shifting silt and sand brought here by the Fraser River. In spring, when the river swelled with melted snow, the island would be flooded and only the tops of the alder and cottonwood trees would stay above water.

About 15 to 20 minutes from the picnic area the trail forks. Go right to follow the Riverside Walk. At first you pass through a marshy area that has skunk cabbage, thimbleberry and more alder and cottonwood. Then the trail breaks into the open and the path is suddenly lined with beach pea, rushes and horsetails (see p. 144) instead.

At the intersection with the Island Tip Trail, continue straight to pass over the George Massey Tunnel (built in 1959) and all the traffic zipping below. Not much farther, a tall channel marker stands on the riverbank. This place is a popular fishing spot and a good tree-free viewpoint from which, on good days, you can see as far as the Gulf Islands and the distant peaks of Vancouver Island.

Black Cottonwood *(Populus balsamifera)*

The black cottonwood (shown in the photo, opposite) is the largest deciduous tree native to BC. It grows very quickly—up to 2 metres (or the height of a tall adult) each year—and it can grow as tall as 50 metres.

The easiest way to identify the black cottonwood is by its heart-shaped leaves and furrowed bark. In late spring it's also easy to identify by its seeds, which come in puffy white clusters that look like tiny cotton balls. When the wind is blowing the seeds around, it can sometimes look like it's snowing.

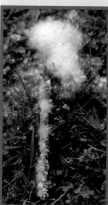

The roots of the black cottonwood help to keep the loose soil of many riverbanks more stable. And, when the leaves fall into the water and decay, they are eaten by many kinds of insects, which in turn are eaten by fish, such as salmon and trout. Other animals also eat parts of the black cottonwood—deer, elk and moose eat its twigs and buds. Beavers eat the inner bark.

In addition, other animals use dead or dying cottonwood trees for shelter. Owls, woodpeckers and bats nest or roost in trees where a big branch or the top of the tree has broken off. Hollow trees often have burrows dug under them by raccoons and black bears.

The trail continues along the riverside to another viewpoint at the southwestern tip of the island, then loops back through the woods to the main trail, over the tunnel and to an intersection. Go right to take the Sand Dune Trail through sand dunes and a grove of shore pine that can make you feel like you're at the seaside. Neither the sand nor the pines came here on their own. The sand was dredged from the river and a scout group planted the trees in the early 1980s.

At the next fork, stay right to take the Dyke Loop Trail, which passes thickets of snowberry shrubs and horsetails.

The path, lined by marsh and the occasional bigleaf maple or cottonwood tree, continues through one of the prettiest parts of the park, called Hawk's Hollow. It gets its name from the red-tailed hawks and Cooper's hawks that you can often see riding the air currents here as they search for a meal.

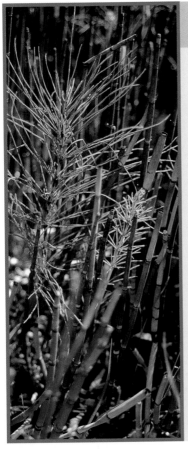

Horsetails
(*Equisetum* spp.)

There are about 20 species of horsetails in the world, about half of which are found in BC. They're among the most primitive forms of plant life. Their ancestors—the much bigger, treelike calamites—arose more than 300 million years ago during the Carboniferous period. (That's about 150 million years before dinosaurs made their appearance.)

Although horsetails prefer moist soil, they can grow just about anywhere. After Mount St. Helen's 1980 volcanic eruption, the first plant seen poking through the debris was the common horsetail.

The common horsetail was once used to prospect for gold. When this species of horsetail grows in soil that has gold in it, it absorbs the gold. People would gather up large amounts of horsetails, burn them and retrieve the gold from the ash. A tonne of stems would contain about 125 grams of gold, worth about $1200 at today's prices.

About 10 to 15 minutes along the Dyke Loop Trail, look for a side trail that branches to the right. It leads to a viewpoint that looks out over Deas Slough, where rowers often practise. You might also see hawks, eagles and owls from here.

Return to the main trail and turn right to continue. Not much farther there is a trail intersection. Continue straight ahead on the Slough View Trail for another 15 minutes or so to reach the Riverside picnic area where you started. (The trail left goes to the Fisher's Field picnic area.)

Cooper's Hawk *(Accipiter cooperii)*

The Cooper's hawk, at 35 to 50 centimetres long, is about the size of a big crow. It is smaller than the red-tailed hawk (55 centimetres long), but bigger than the sharp-shinned hawk (30 centimetres long), which it resembles. It is coloured blue-grey above and light below, with reddish-brown barring.

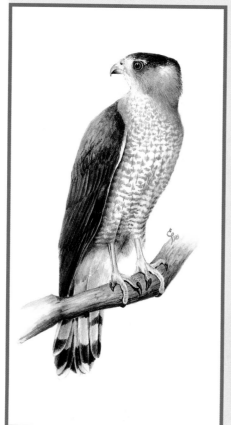

The *Accipiter* genus, to which both the Cooper's and sharp-shinned hawks belong, is a group of hawks with long tails and short, rounded wings that give these birds tremendous flying agility.

This small hawk hunts by flying low over the trees, using them to hide itself from its prey. It preys mostly on songbirds, although it will also take squirrels, chipmunks, frogs and even an occasional barnyard chicken. You might also see a Cooper's hawk hanging out near a backyard feeder, where the chances are good for finding a songbird meal.

The Cooper's hawk builds its nest at least 10 metres up in a tree, using twigs that it breaks off in an unusual manner. While in flight, the hawk grasps a twig with its feet and uses its momentum to snap it from the branch.

Brunswick Point

Length: 5 km

Time needed: 2 to 2.5 hours

Season: Year-round

Rating: Easy

Dogs: Yes, on leash

Stroller-friendly: Yes

Washrooms: None

Highlights: Old cannery, marshland, dykes, winter birds

Access: Follow Highway 99 south to Ladner, taking exit 28 (the Tsawwassen and Ferries exit) southbound. Follow Highway 17 to Ladner Trunk Road (the first traffic lights) and turn right. Continue on Ladner Trunk Road (it turns into 47A Avenue just past Ladner's town centre) to River Road West. Follow River Road past the turn-off for the Reifel Migratory Bird Sanctuary, and park at the end of the road. Do not block any driveways.

Driving time: 45 minutes

Dykes protect low-lying farmlands from being flooded by the sea. But they're also great places for people to walk, bicycle and ride horses. The dykes of Brunswick Point have some of the prettiest surroundings, including marshes and farmland. On clear days you can also enjoy views of the distant mountains.

From the road, head for the top of the dyke. This part of the dyke shadows Canoe Passage, the skinny little arm of the Fraser River that separates Westham Island from the mainland. Because the passage is so narrow, tidal action can make the water really scoot through it at times. Harbour seals, ducks and gulls bobbing on the currents can look like they're zipping along on a long conveyor belt.

After the remains of an old farmhouse on the left, there's a marshy section on the right that has rows and rows of old pilings. These pilings are all that's left of the old Brunswick Cannery.

Brunswick Point dykes

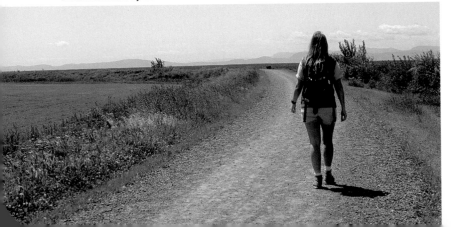

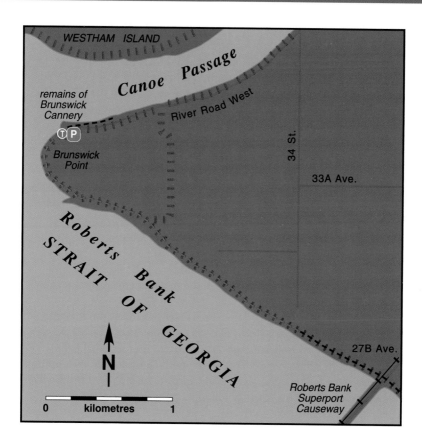

The Cannery

The Brunswick Cannery was one of 14 canneries that operated in Delta in the 1870s and 1880s. Canoe Passage was wider and deeper then. And there were many more salmon than there are today—a single night's catch in the area was counted at 75,000 salmon.

In the 1890s, though, there were a lot of floods in this part of the Fraser. Silt began to build up, narrowing Canoe Passage, and few salmon swam through anymore. So the canning industry eventually shut down.

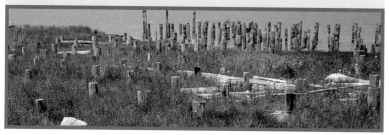

Although the silt was detrimental to the salmon (see p. 147), one positive result was that it made more marsh—important habitat for all kinds of wild animals. If you're here in springtime, you'll see bright yellow flowers in the marsh. Although its flowers are pretty, the yellow flag iris is not native to BC and is not as important to the creatures of the marsh as the native plants are.

Continue along the dyke as it curves southwest. If you had walked here about 100 years ago, you'd have been at least knee-deep in water or marsh, because the dykes weren't here yet.

Continue farther south along the dyke trail to see where a row of trees was planted long ago as a windbreak. In at least two of the trees, bald eagles have built nests. (Red-tailed hawks built the nests first but were elbowed out by the eagles, which then built bigger nests.)

There's a wealth of bird life here. Probably the best time to see it is in winter. On the tidal flats there are big flocks of shorebirds, including sandpipers, sanderlings and dunlin. In the marsh there are swans, snow geese and snowy owls.

After you've passed the last farm, you will see 34th Street on the other side of a deep, uncrossable ditch. The dyke continues farther—all the way to (and beyond) the Roberts Bank jetty, where trains carry coal to be loaded onto freighters bound for foreign ports. This is a good turn-around point, so retrace your steps, once again taking in the beauty of Brunswick Point, this time with the North Shore mountains as a backdrop.

Transient & Overwintering Birds

Many shorebirds, along with snowy owls (illustrated), trumpeter swans and snow geese, spend summers building nests and raising their young in places farther north. In winter, though, when it's too cold for them to hang out on 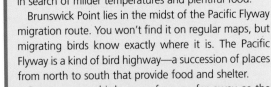 the arctic tundra or in the BC Interior, they migrate south in search of milder temperatures and plentiful food.

Brunswick Point lies in the midst of the Pacific Flyway migration route. You won't find it on regular maps, but migrating birds know exactly where it is. The Pacific Flyway is a kind of bird highway—a succession of places from north to south that provide food and shelter.

Because some birds come from as far away as the Arctic, they need to make several pit stops on their journeys south to rest and refuel (with food). Each spring and autumn, hundreds of different bird species pass through or over Brunswick Point—one of the stops on the Pacific Flyway. Some birds, called transients, stay for just a few weeks; others stay the whole winter.

The Value of Marshland

Marsh plants supply food and shelter for many different animals. The red-winged blackbird and the marsh wren use cattails to perch on and to build their nests in. Ducks and geese feed on the roots and shoots in the marsh. Field mice and Townsend's voles scurry among the sedges and grasses. Hawks and owls prey on the mice and voles, keeping the rodent population in check.

A marsh, in this case a salt-marsh, is a kind of wetland. Wetlands are basically soggy places—some are soggy year-round, and others may dry out during the hottest, driest days of summer.

Think of a wetland as a kind of biological supermarket. In one aisle, you've got dead plants that break down and provide food for insects, shellfish and small fish. In the next aisle, those same insects, shellfish and small fish are available to be gobbled up by frogs, bigger fish, snakes, birds and mammals.

If a wetland is destroyed, all the creatures that depend on it for food and shelter can also be destroyed.

Dyking the Fraser River Delta

Much of the Lower Mainland is built on the delta of the Fraser River. A delta is the land that gets built up where a river meets the sea and drops the silt and sand and gravel that it has carried.

Over the years, all the material washed downstream has built up to become a substantial mass of land in the midst of the Fraser River. However, it remains lowland and therefore subject to flooding each spring when rain and melting snow in the mountains cause the river to rise.

When settlers started to move into the lower parts of the Lower Mainland to farm, the yearly floods would often inundate their farms, fields and crops. So, beginning in 1895, they built a system of dykes to protect their properties. The dykes have changed the terrain of the delta, but wildlife has adapted to most of the changes. In the areas that once were marsh but now are fields, you'll see hawks and owls patrolling for mice and other rodents.

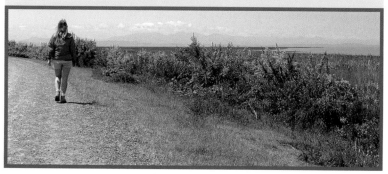

Reifel Migratory Bird Sanctuary

Length: 3-km loop

Time needed: 1.5 to 2 hours

Season: Year-round

Rating: Easy

Dogs: No

Stroller-friendly: All-terrain stroller only

Washrooms: In parking area

Highlights: Bird blinds, observation tower, migrating birds

Access: Follow Highway 99 south to Ladner, taking exit 28 (the Tsawwassen and Ferries exit) southbound. Follow Highway 17 to Ladner Trunk Road (the first traffic light) and turn right. Continue on Ladner Trunk Road (it turns into 47A Avenue just past Ladner's town centre) to River Road West. At Westham Island Road, go right and over the single-lane wooden bridge. Follow Westham Island Road (which becomes Robertson Road) to its end and go left to enter the sanctuary, following that road to its end. Park.

Note: Entrance fee required.

Driving time: 45 minutes

Reifel Migratory Bird Sanctuary is a Lower Mainland mecca for birders of all ages and abilities. Even if you're not a birding buff, Reifel is a lovely destination for a walk on wooded and dyke-top paths. It's as much a sanctuary for people as it is for birds.

Before you even get out of the car, you'll see birds. The usual mallards and Canada geese hang out in the ponds adjacent to the parking area, always happy for a handout of bird food. Roosters can be seen crowing and strutting in the grassy area to the west. If you're lucky, a resident sandhill crane with its bright red cap and lanky legs may stride through the parking area.

Head to the main gate and pay the entrance fee ($4 for adults, $2 for kids aged 2 to 14 and $2 for seniors). Another 50¢ will buy a bag of bird food. (Don't feed bread to birds because it has almost no nutritional value for them.)

Migratory bird habitat

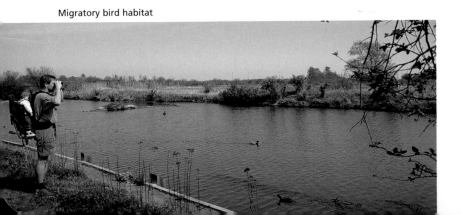

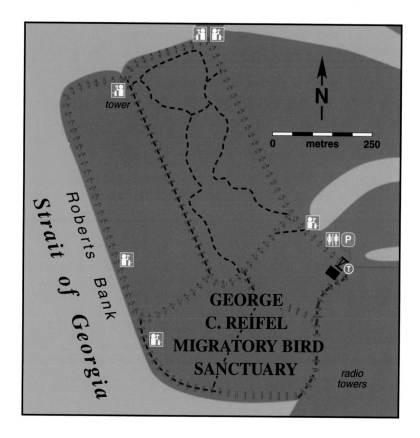

Once through the gate, stop just around the building's corner for a look at which notable bird species have been seen in the sanctuary recently. About 100 metres from the entrance there are information signs that tell more about the kinds of birds here during the different seasons, and about estuaries, snow geese and what the area looked like years ago before it was a sanctuary.

Continue straight ahead, past a small pond and along a dyke path lined with Douglas-fir trees. Walk quietly and you can expect to see lots of small birds foraging along the path.

In spring, summer or autumn, up to six species of swallow fly over the fields in this area in search of insects. And, if you look carefully among the branches of the Douglas-fir trees that you pass, you might spot one of the eight species of owls seen in the sanctuary.

At the end of the path, go right and follow a side trail that leads to a blind from where you can watch the birds.

Return to the main trail and go right again to another blind. This blind looks out onto salt-marsh. You'll usually see red-winged blackbirds here.

Using a Blind

When you're in a blind, it's important to be quiet. The purpose of a blind is for you to hide from the birds so that they don't know that you're there watching them. That way you get to see ducks, geese, herons (illustrated) and other birds that aren't comfortable having people around.

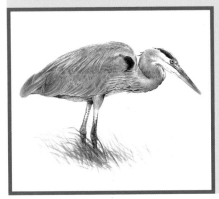

Birders and ornithologists (bird scientists) use blinds to watch the behaviour of birds. Photographers use blinds to get better pictures of birds.

Although blinds are now often used by people who want to watch birds without disturbing or harming them, they were first used (and still are) by hunters to allow them to get close enough to birds to shoot them.

But, depending on the season, you might also see swans, snow geese and other waterfowl. Look to the row of conifers in the distance and you might also see a bald eagle.

Return to the main trail again and go right. A few minutes of walking brings you to an observation tower. Go up and take a look. From the top of the tower there is a great view of the salt-marsh that surrounds the paths and ponds of the sanctuary. You can also see Roberts Bank and Point Roberts, USA, to the south, and beyond that, some of the Gulf Islands and San Juan Islands. To the north is the Sunshine Coast.

Return to the T junction and go left to follow the trail around the perimeter of the ponds. This wide, open path allows a better look at some of the shorebirds and waterfowl that spend time in these ponds. The types and abundance of shorebirds vary with the season. In winter, there are almost no shorebirds; in spring, the ponds are packed with a variety of species.

About halfway down the dyke you'll come across another blind. A bit farther along there is a wooden platform and a bench that marks a trail junction. Go left to wander along more ponds and sloughs. At the next T junction, go right. Another wooden platform gives you a better look at some of the pond inhabitants.

The trail then returns to a slightly wooded section. In summer, an arch of green foliage frames the trail. Continue straight and you will arrive back at the intersection where you started. Go right to return to the sanctuary entrance.

Shorebirds & Seasons

Shorebirds are small wading birds that forage along sandy beaches, mud-flats and estuaries for tiny crustaceans, aquatic insects and worms.

These birds vary in size from tiny least sandpipers about the size of a house sparrow to greater yellowlegs that are just a bit smaller than our northwestern crow. Their bills are usually quite slender, but they may vary in length from just a centimetre to more than 20 centimetres. That allows different species to probe the mud and sand at different levels.

Here at Reifel, certain species, such as the killdeer and the western sandpiper, reside year-round. But others, such as the dunlin, the greater yellowlegs and the long-billed dowitcher, are usually seen only during the spring or autumn migration. (Reifel lies on the Pacific Flyway, a kind of bird superhighway that stretches from northern Canada, Alaska and Siberia to South America.)

Spring is probably the best time to see shorebirds en masse at Reifel: more than one million shorebirds can be seen on a single day.

Reifel dyke trail

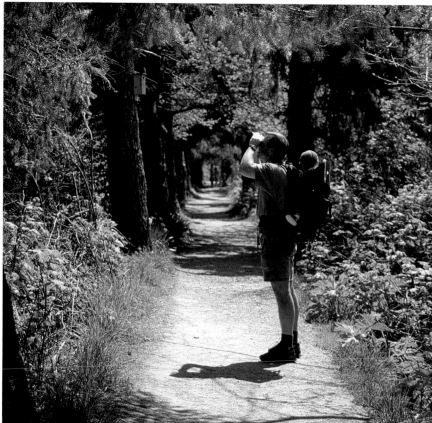

Boundary Bay

Length: 4 km

Time needed: 2 to 2.5 hours

Season: Year-round

Rating: Easy

Dogs: Yes, on leash

Stroller-friendly: Yes

Washrooms: Outhouse at Delta Air Park

Highlights: Tansy, red-tailed hawks, great blue herons, oyster plant relics

Access: Take Highway 99 south to exit 20 (North Delta, Surrey). Go straight at the stoplight. As the road veers left, it becomes Hornby Drive. Follow it to 104th Street. Turn right and go past the Delta Air Park to the dyke entrance. Parking is limited.

Driving time: 35 minutes

Boundary Bay is a favourite with walkers, cyclists and horseback riders. With more than 16 kilometres of dykes stretching from Beach Grove to Mud Bay and lots of access points, there are many different sections to walk. My favourite section begins here, at the south end of 104th Street.

Before you start walking on the dyke, take a look at the plane parked right near the entrance gate to the Delta Air Park. It's a Lockheed Lodestar built in 1940 by Trans Canada Airways. Then head back to the trailhead at the dyke.

Once on top of the dyke, go left and through the gate. If you're here in summer, there will be many kinds of wildflowers along both sides of the dyke path, including the orange-red blossoms of fireweed, the big pink blooms of common vetch, the white blossoms of blackberry and the sunny yellow flowers of common tansy.

Common tansy

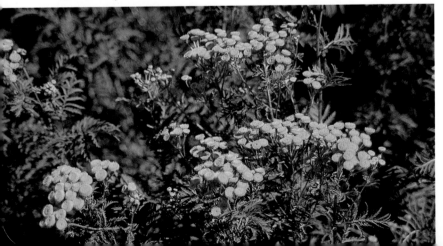

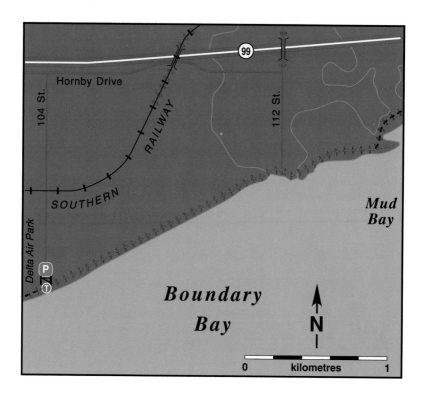

Common Tansy *(Tanacetum vulgare)*

Two species of tansy grow in BC: dune tansy *(Tanacetum bipinnatum)* grows on sand dunes; common tansy grows along roadsides and railways and in other disturbed habitats. Both species of tansy look alike with their clusters of button-shaped, yellow flowers.

One important difference between the two species is that dune tansy is native to BC while common tansy is native to Great Britain. When common tansy arrived in BC, it started as a plant in people's gardens. Seeds may have drifted from gardens to fields or someone may have dumped some old plants by the roadside, and suddenly common tansy was growing all over the place.

It sounds like a good thing—more wildflowers to look at, right? But there can be problems when non-native plants such as tansy get out of the garden. If they are fast growers, they can take over places that used to be occupied by native plants.

Further problems can develop if, for instance, a particular kind of insect, bird or mammal depends on a certain native plant for food or shelter. If it becomes scarce because a non-native plant has been replacing it, then there is going to be less food or shelter available for that insect, bird or animal, and so it too will become scarce.

As you continue along the dyke trail, keep your eyes to the skies, especially the skies above the fields on the left. If you're lucky you'll see hawks as they swoop and soar looking for mice and other little rodents to eat.

Red-tailed Hawk *(Buteo jamaicensis)*

The red-tailed hawk, which is slightly larger than a crow, is often seen near Boundary Bay. What are some of the clues that can help you tell this hawk from others? If the bird is close enough and the lighting is right, the reddish tailfeathers are a good clue. Most red-tailed hawks also have a white chest

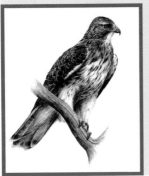

and what birders call a speckled 'belly-band' that can make it look as if the hawk is wearing a wide, speckled belt around its belly.

Otherwise, red-tailed hawks vary a lot in their coloration. They can be reddish-brown all over or almost all grey or a pale brown and white.

The other noticeable thing about a red-tailed hawk is how it often hovers in one place while looking for food. This hawk eats mice, rats and other rodents, as well as the occasional snake or small bird.

Oyster-shucking Plant

More than 100 years ago, an oyster plant was built here on Boundary Bay. There were so many oysters back then that oyster gatherers would harvest 35,000 oysters at a time. Then they took the oysters to the oyster plant and the workers there would shuck them (remove the edible parts from the shell).

After just 20 years of such harvests, all the native oysters were pretty much gone. Not ready to give up, oyster merchants brought in a different species of oyster, the Atlantic oyster, which is native to the Atlantic Ocean. That strategy allowed the oyster business to last until the 1930s.

Then, in 1941, oyster operators introduced more than 4 million Japanese oysters to the bay. The oyster business continued until 1961 when the plant was shut down and, later, torn down. By then the bay's waters had become so polluted that it was no longer safe to eat the oysters—or the mussels, clams and crabs—that lived in Boundary Bay.

These days, the Department of Fisheries and Oceans regulates the harvest of shellfish. Some, such as oysters, can't be harvested at all in the Lower Mainland. For others, such as clams and crabs, there are rules about when you can get them, how many you can take and how big they have to be.

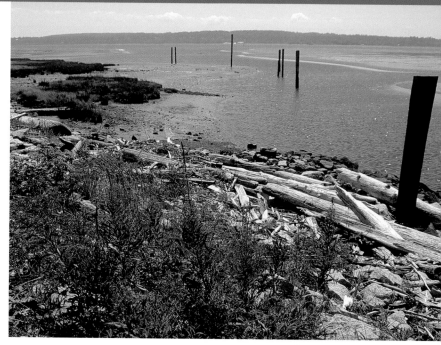

Pilings at Boundary Bay

Where the dyke trail starts to curve left, look on the right for a side trail that leads through the grass. Follow it toward a group of trees, keeping an eye out for little songbirds that flit and fly around here. Then follow it a bit farther to where the trail finally ends at the edge of a tidal marsh.

You can see several different species of sedges and grasses growing here. And there's lots of driftwood and other bits of stuff, brought here during the highest tides of winter. After a good look around, retrace your steps to the dyke trail again.

Turn left and head back east. On the return trip, focus your attention on the bay side of the trail. Across the bay is Tsawwassen and the community of Beach Grove.

In Boundary Bay, the water is very shallow, because of all the silt and sediment that gets brought in by the creeks and rivers that drain into it. When the tide is low, you can see wide mud-flats (or tidal flats) that stretch for a very long way. Although they may not look very lush, these tidal flats provide lots of food for many different creatures, especially birds.

Continue along the dyke trail back toward the gate. Notice the old pilings sticking out of the mud. They're all that's left of some buildings that used to perch here on the flats (see p. 156).

Once you're back at the gate, you can return to your car. Or, if you want to wander farther, you can keep walking more of the dyke trail.

Burns Bog (Delta Nature Reserve)

Length: 4-km loop
Time needed: 2 to 2.5 hours
Season: Year-round
Rating: Easy
Dogs: Yes, on leash
Stroller-friendly: All-terrain stroller only
Washrooms: None
Highlights: Bog-laurel, wildlife trails, shore pine, buried bulldozer

Access: Take Highway 91 southbound over the Alex Fraser Bridge. Then take the first exit (Nordel Way, River Road). Stay right as if going to River Road and continue through the first set of traffic lights. At the next set of lights, go right onto Nordel Court and follow the road to the Great Pacific Forum. Park at the far end of the parking lot.

Driving time: 30 minutes

Hikes along rivers, through forests or up mountains are popular with many people. But a hike through a bog? Most people think that it would mean trudging through a lot of mud and muck. But they'd be wrong. This hike through part of Burns Bog shows just how nice a walk through the bog can be.

Burns Bog Wildlife

Even though Burns Bog is close to urban areas, lots of animals still live here because they can find both food and shelter in the bog.

Some of the animal trails that you see may have been made by black-tailed (mule) deer, which feed on plants such as salal, huckleberry and western redcedar. Other trails might have been made by coyotes, which eat the mice, shrews, squirrels and frogs that are also found here.

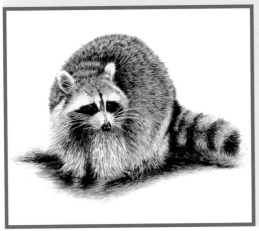

Although they are very rarely seen, black bears also live in Burns Bog (although probably not in this part of the bog). Other mammals you might spot are raccoons, beavers, muskrats, skunks, porcupines, red foxes and bobcats.

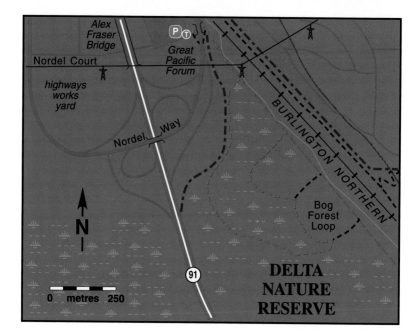

The hike starts just past the chain-link fence at the east end of the parking lot. Look for the brick cyclist and pedestrian path and go left under the overpass. Once on the other side, follow the short brick-paved jog left that brings you to a gravel road. You'll soon see a blue sign that indicates the boundary of the Delta Nature Reserve. On the left is a wooden bench. A tiny creek trickles just behind it.

Continue along the gravel road, enjoying the dapples of sun and shade created by the alder and cottonwood trees on both sides. Within 10 minutes or less, you come to a towering power pylon. Just past it, on the right, is the start of a boardwalk trail. Go right through a bit of mixed forest to emerge into the bog proper.

Where the boardwalk ends, continue straight ahead along the trail. Almost immediately, you'll notice how springy the ground under your feet is. That's because it's not just dirt beneath your boots—it's metres and metres of peat. (Peat is made up of dead and decaying plant matter.) The trail is lined on both sides by shrubs such as Labrador tea and western bog-laurel (see p. 161).

As you continue along the trail, notice all the tiny side trails that jut off the main trail. These trails are used by some of the animals that live in and around the bog.

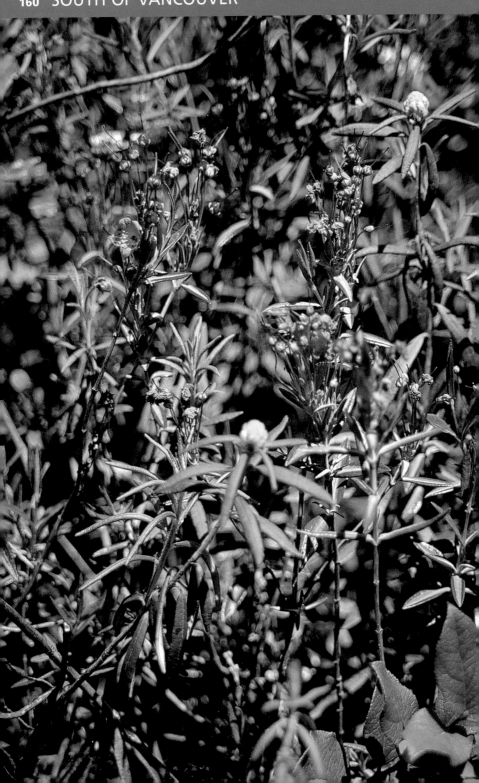

Western Bog-laurel *(Kalmia microphylla)*

Western bog-laurel (shown in photo, opposite) is easiest to recognize in spring, when it is in bloom with pretty saucer-shaped pink flowers.

If you look closely, you'll see what look like 10 tiny little flagpoles inside the flower. These are called stamens; the anthers at their tips make the flower's pollen. The stamens are meant to be triggered by insects, who will then carry the pollen to another western bog-laurel flower and transfer the pollen to a part of the flower called the stigma. It sits on top of the pistil—the white stalk in the centre of the flower that produces the seeds. Later, when the flower falls off, the seed capsule is left behind. Although it looks like a bright red berry, it is poisonous and should not be eaten.

Warning: Although western bog-laurel is a pretty plant, it is also poisonous. Never eat or taste any part of the plant.

As you continue along the trail, you may find the ground getting a bit wetter and mushier, especially if it's been raining or if it's wintertime. Sections of boardwalk help you over the wettest parts and eventually bring you to a fork in the trail.

Go left. You soon come to more boardwalk. The shrubs on either side of the trail here, such as hardhack, are slightly different from those you've seen so far. In spring, hardhack has conical clusters of pink blossoms; the rest of the year you can see the dead brown flower husks. There is also Pacific crabapple, BC's only native apple tree. It's easy to recognize in spring by its sweet-scented white to pink blossoms and in autumn by its tiny apples.

You're soon walking on bog again. Now is the time to start really noticing what species of trees are along the trail. Although you might see an occasional western hemlock or western redcedar, most of the trees here are still shore pines. The spongy ground under your feet shares an important characteristic with the trees that surround you—they both remove carbon dioxide from the atmosphere (see p. 162).

For a while, the trail is tangled with roots and can often be wet. Soon, though, it enters forest again. Notice how the understorey changes from bog shrubs to a mixture of bog shrubs and forest plants and then finally to a relatively bare forest floor. The trees here are mostly hemlock and redcedar. They offer cool shade on hot days.

For the next 20 minutes or so, the trail wanders in and out through slightly different types of forest: open forest with ferns and salmonberries, mixed forest with alder and Sitka spruce trees, then back into the cool, dark stands of hemlock and cedar.

You're soon back in the sunlight and a marshy bog section. Then, back into the forest again. About 30 metres ahead is a trail junction. Go left.

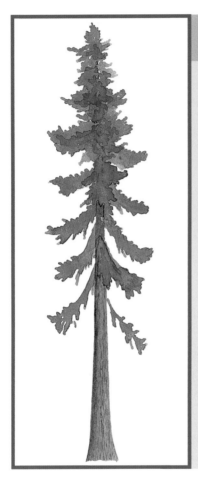

Trees, Bogs & Carbon Dioxide

Carbon dioxide constitutes only 0.03 percent of our atmosphere, but it plays an important role in regulating temperature on the planet. Without it, the earth would be a much colder place. But if there is too much carbon dioxide, temperatures rise, with a variety of effects on climate, sea level and weather. It's a phenomenon known as global warming.

Both trees (such as western redcedar, illustrated) and bogs play an important role in reducing the amount of carbon dioxide in the atmosphere. Trees absorb carbon dioxide from the air in the process of photosynthesis and use the carbon as fuel. Bogs also absorb carbon dioxide from the air, then store the carbon as peat.

Trees and bogs play an important role in helping to slow global warming. The concern is that when forests are cut or when peatlands are disturbed, carbon is released, contributing to the acceleration of global warming.

Not much farther along is another length of boardwalk that takes you past huge skunk cabbage, salal and more Pacific crabapple.

Another 10 minutes or so of walking brings you to another trail junction. Stay left. Not much farther ahead, look on the left for a side trail that leads to a small clearing and a bench. It's a nice place for a break and maybe a snack.

Back on the main trail, continue for another few minutes to reach another boardwalk section and a platform with benches all around. They provide a perfect viewpoint from which to look at a bulldozer mired in the bog.

Continue along the boardwalk for a few minutes more to come back to the service road. Go left, toward the power pylon. You will pass the trail on which you started. Continue straight ahead to return to the parking lot via the brick pathway.

The Buried Bulldozer

Although it might look as if it's been here forever, this bulldozer has been in the bog for only a few years. It was stolen from a construction site nearby and driven into the bog. After a day, it had already sunk way down into the peat. When initial efforts to retrieve it were unsuccessful, no one bothered to try again. It has since become a point of interest for visitors to the park.

Buried bulldozer

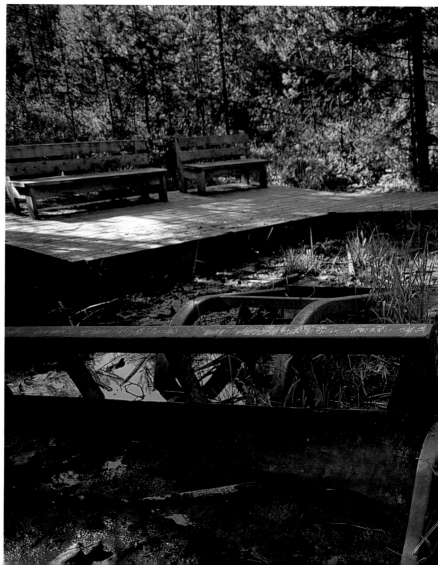

Serpentine Fen

Length: 4.5-km loop

Time needed: 2 to 2.5 hours

Season: Year-round

Rating: Easy

Dogs: No

Stroller-friendly: All-terrain stroller only

Washrooms: None

Highlights: Observation tower, ducks, northern harriers, Serpentine River

Access: Take Highway 99 southbound to exit 10 (White Rock, Crescent Beach). Go right toward Crescent Beach, but then steer left onto Nicomekl Road. At King George Highway (Highway 99A), go left again. Pass over the freeway and look for the Wildlife Viewing sign. Just past Art Knapp Plantland, turn left onto 44th Avenue. Pass the yellow gate and go along the bumpy road. At the orange gate, go left into the parking lot.

Driving time: 45 minutes

Nestled between two highways, Serpentine Fen may not seem like the most attractive place to go for a walk among nature's beauty. But when you're there ambling along the dyke trails, it's easy to forget the traffic.

From the parking lot, walk back to the orange gate, pass it and head up the dirt road. At the end of the road, cross a little bridge to the observation tower. From the top of the tower, there's a good view of most of Serpentine Fen—its marsh, ponds, fields and hedgerows.

Serpentine wetland

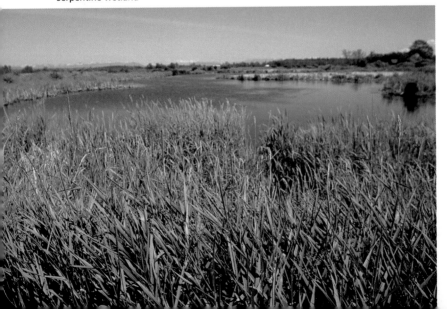

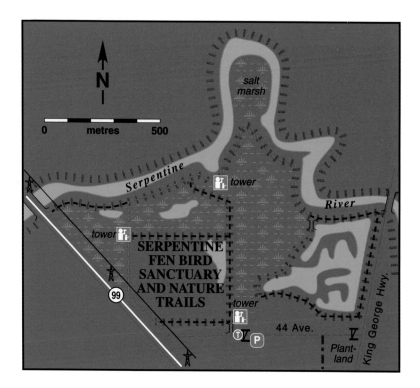

Go back down the tower stairs and follow the path along the wire fence. The path leads to several dykes. Although some areas are closed to provide quieter habitat for the resident species, you can follow the open dyke between the ponds.

Ducks

The duck that most people know best is the mallard. But there are lots of other kinds of ducks. The mallard is a dabbling duck, and so are the green-winged teal and the northern pintail. Dabbling ducks bob about, their tails above the water, as they dabble for plants, seeds and water snails. Other dabblers you might see at Serpentine Fen include the northern shoveler and the American widgeon. Diving ducks, on the other hand, dive down under the water to look for fish, mussels, crabs and aquatic insects. Some diving ducks that you might see here include buffleheads (illustrated) and common mergansers.

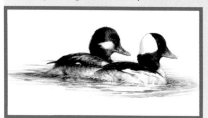

In the course of the year, about 175 species of birds—including shore-birds, waterfowl, birds of prey and songbirds—come to Serpentine Fen for food, shelter or nesting sites. In spring, summer and autumn, swallows swoop down, skimming the surfaces of ponds in their search for insects. Red-winged blackbirds often cling to the cattails, chortling their familiar *konk-a-ree* call. Great blue herons stalk the shallows looking for small fish or frogs to eat.

If you look above the marshes and fields, you might see another frequent visitor, a bird of prey called the northern harrier.

Eventually, the dyke trail leads to a small bridge. Cross it to come to the Serpentine River. Go left on the wide dyke trail here. On the left you may notice some plants with little blue or yellow flags attached to them. They are part of a Wildlife Enhancement Program (a collaborative project between government and non-profit organizations) that will add to the number of native trees and shrubs in the area in order to provide more habitat for raptors (birds of prey) and songbirds.

A short distance farther along the trail will bring you to a small island. Look at the mud banks and you might see some burrows that muskrats have dug. After walking about 10 minutes longer, you will arrive at the second observation tower. Climb up for a better look at the Serpentine River.

Northern Harrier *(Circus cyaneus)*

The northern harrier frequents marsh and field habitats because that's where it finds mice, rats, birds, frogs, snakes and other small animals to eat. In some parts of North America, this bird is known as a 'marsh hawk' because of its preference for marshes; it even builds its nests in the marshes. First the harrier makes a hollow in the ground, then it makes a nest of small sticks, reeds and

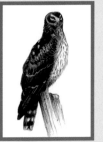

grasses. The nest, which is usually hidden in the brush, can be as big as a metre across.

About the same size as a red-tailed hawk, the northern harrier has a longer tail and longer wings. The male is grey on top and white below, and the female is brown on top and streaky brown below. The face of a northern harrier looks a little different from that of most hawks because its eyes are set in shallow, disk-like hollows, like an owl's eyes are. Biologists believe that this shape might let harriers focus sound better than other hawks do, so that they can better hear a mouse or bird rustling in the grass.

The northern harrier hunts by flying close to the ground and then swooping down quickly on its prey. The best time to see the northern harrier is at dusk, its preferred time to hunt.

Go back down the stairs and continue westward. Some old pilings stand here. Look over the dyke to the water's low-tide line and you'll see oyster shells, proof that salt water from Mud Bay mixes with the river's fresh water.

You will then come to a trail that leads left off the main dyke. Follow it toward the third observation tower. (The main dyke trail ends a bit farther ahead at Highway 99.) From the top of the third tower you can see more ponds that are often full of a variety of different waterfowl, including many kinds of ducks (see p. 165).

Head back down the tower stairs for the last stretch of trail. This section goes under giant power pylons and parallels Highway 99. It can be noisy, and it certainly isn't the best part of Serpentine Fen, but you can often see lots of little songbirds here. Soon you will be back at the road that you came in on. Retrace your steps to the parking lot and picnic area.

The Serpentine River

From the top of the tower you can see how the river gets its name. Don't all the twists and turns in the river remind you of a serpent or a snake?

The Serpentine River makes a lot of twists and turns on its way from its headwaters in north Surrey's Tynehead Park to where it empties into Mud Bay, but the most winding and wiggling part can be seen from the observation tower.

The river is always changing its course by eroding its banks in one place and adding to them somewhere else, but the process usually happens too slowly to be noticed. Higher-than-normal water levels rushing down a river can cut through a bank much more dramatically, and that's what has happened just east of the observation tower. A chunk of the old bank now sits in the middle of the river like a little island.

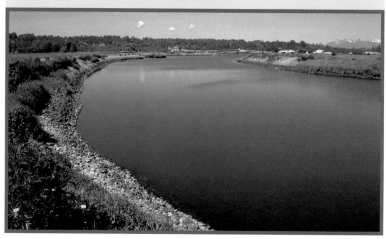

Blackie Spit

Length: 5-km loop

Time needed: 2 to 2.5 hours

Season: Year-round

Rating: Easy

Dogs: Yes, on leash

Stroller-friendly: No

Washrooms: In trailer in parking lot at Blackie Spit

Highlights: Shellfish, overwintering birds, salt-marsh, sea asparagus

Access: Head southward on Highway 99 and take the Crescent Beach turn-off. Bear right to follow Nicomekl Road over a narrow bridge that is actually the top of a dam. Turn right onto Crescent Road and follow it for about 5 kilometres, turning right onto Sullivan Street just past the railway tracks. At McBride Avenue, go right again to the parking lot at Blackie Spit Park.

Driving time: 1 hour

Head to the waterfront for views across Boundary Bay to Tsawwassen and Point Roberts. From autumn until early spring there are big flocks of ducks bobbing on the waves.

Now head for the beach. Walk eastward along the sand. There are lots of different shells—clams, mussels, cockles—but oyster shells, either whole or in broken bits, are the most plentiful.

Shellfish

Archaeologists believe that the Coast Salish people gathered shellfish at Blackie Spit as long ago as 8000 years.

Some of the shells on the beach are different from those that were here 100 years ago. That's because people in the shellfish industry brought shellfish here from other places in the world, usually because they were bigger and had more meat or because they grew faster than the native species.

Although the shellfish industry benefited from the introduction of new species to the area, it was not a good thing for the native species of shellfish. For example, when Japanese oysters were introduced to BC, a serious oyster pest, the Japanese oyster drill, was also accidentally introduced. Not only did it harm the Japanese oysters, it also attacked our native oyster species.

These days, the harvesting of clams, oysters, cockles and mussels in Boundary Bay and Mud Bay is banned because of pollution.

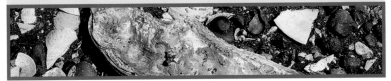

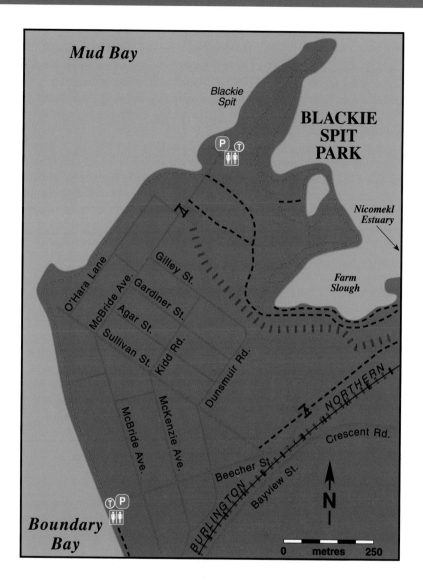

Mud Bay

Blackie
Spit

**BLACKIE
SPIT
PARK**

Nicomekl
Estuary

Farm
Slough

O'Hara Lane

McBride Ave.

Gardiner St.

Gilley St.

Agar St.

Sullivan St.

Kidd Rd.

Dunsmuir Rd.

McBride Ave.

McKenzie Ave.

NORTHERN

Crescent Rd.

Beecher St.

Bayview St.

BURLINGTON

*Boundary
Bay*

N

0   metres   250

Overwintering Ducks

Although some birds live in the Lower Mainland all year, others spend their summers feeding and nesting farther north and spend only their winters here.

Among the birds that overwinter here in big flocks are the surf scoter, American widgeon, greater and lesser scaup and Barrow's goldeneye. Use binoculars and a good field guide, such as *Birds of Coastal British Columbia*, to help identify the different kinds of ducks.

Continue walking around Blackie Spit—named after Walter Blackie, who lived and farmed here in the late 1800s—toward where the Nicomekl River spills into Mud Bay. This place, where the river meets the sea, is called a river estuary. As you come around the tip of the spit, notice the wide flats of mud with plants growing on it. This part of the estuary is called a salt-marsh (see p. 171).

It's best to stay off the flats—to avoid disturbing the birds and to keep from sinking into the mud—and keep on the trail as you try to pick out all the different birds. Maybe you'll see a horned grebe with its eerie red eyes, a green-winged teal with its streak of bright green on its copper-coloured head or a great blue heron stalking a fish.

Stay left between the fence and the water to pick up a trail through a fence opening. Here, in a field among red alder trees and broom bushes, you can see a variety of songbirds and raptors, including red-tailed hawks, northern harriers and bald eagles.

How much of the area you can comfortably explore depends on how wet the field is and what kind of shoes you're wearing. If you can, go toward the water to a narrow trail that runs on top of a small dyke. Soon, the trail drops down. Go left to a small beach where there's a great view.

You soon come to a point where you can go right and walk toward the railway bridge and marina. Take a look at the short stubby plants growing closest to the water. One of them is called sea asparagus (see p. 171).

Continuing along the beach you'll approach a group of old pilings sticking up out of the water. They are all that's left of the old Olympic Oyster Company that used to be here in the 1910s and 1920s. If it's sunny, you might see cormorants perched on the pilings.

Blackie Spit

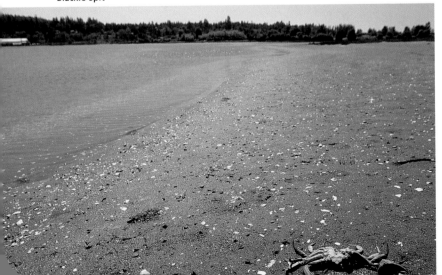

Salt-marshes

As recently as 100 years ago, you could find salt-marshes all along the seashore in the Lower Mainland. But then people built marinas, ferry jetties, coal ports, pulp mills and houses near the water, and many salt-marshes were covered over, filled in or dredged.

In places where salt-marshes survived, many kinds of wildlife flourish. They range from tiny marine creatures and fish to birds and other animals that depend on the smaller creatures and plants for food. Between September and March you can see as many as 200 species of birds here.

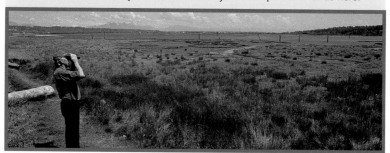

Follow the path back towards Crescent Beach for about 10 minutes. At the trail junction go left and take the narrow trail that leads into the woods on another dyke top. People have hung feeders here that attract songbirds such as finches and towhees.

The trail loops back on top of an open dyke, but first walk past the gate to a point where you can stop for a snack or look at the birds, river and mountains. Then return on the trail to the parking lot where you started.

Sea Asparagus *(Salicornia virginica)*

Look for a plant that resembles a bunch of short, green worms. (In autumn and winter, it may be more purple-brown in colour.) If you break a piece off, you'll notice that it is crunchy. If you wash a tiny piece off and chew it, you'll notice that it's salty and tastes like asparagus. That's why many people call it

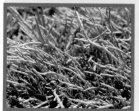 sea asparagus. It's also called saltwort ('wort' is an old English word that means 'plant') or glasswort (referring to the way people used to burn the plant and use the ashes in making glass).

Some people like to eat sea asparagus as a vegetable. The next time you're at Granville Island Market, you might see it for sale.

Redwood Park

Length: 2.5-km loop

Time needed: 1 to 1.5 hours

Season: Year-round

Rating: Easy

Dogs: Yes, on leash

Stroller-friendly: All-terrain stroller only

Washrooms: Near parking area

Highlights: Tree house, giant sequoia trees, woodpeckers, buttercups

Access: Follow Highway 99 south to exit 10 (White Rock, Crescent Beach) and follow it left to King George Highway (Highway 99A). There, go right. At 16th Avenue, turn left and follow the road to 176th Street. Turn left. Drive to 20th Avenue and turn right. About 0.7 kilometres farther is the entrance to Redwood Park. Follow the gravel road to the parking area.

Driving time: 50 minutes

This small park is home to trees and plants that you're used to seeing in southwestern BC forests, but it's also home to some exotic species—such as the giant sequoia—that were planted here almost 100 years ago. There are lots of short trails, as well as open meadow areas in which to picnic and play.

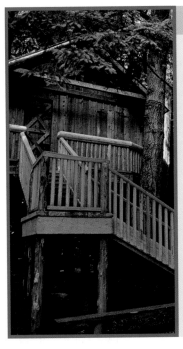

The Tree House

The land that makes up Redwood Park was once part of the homestead of a Surrey pioneer named David Brown. In 1878 he travelled by covered wagon from the eastern US to San Francisco, where he caught a boat to Bellingham. From there, he canoed north to Ferndale, Washington, and then walked the rest of the way here.

When his twin sons David Jr. and Peter turned 21, he gave them each 16 hectares of logged land, which they replanted with trees from around the world. They built a tree house here in 1893 and lived in it until 1958. The tree house that is here today is a replacement of the one the brothers lived in. The original tree house became dilapidated and was torn down.

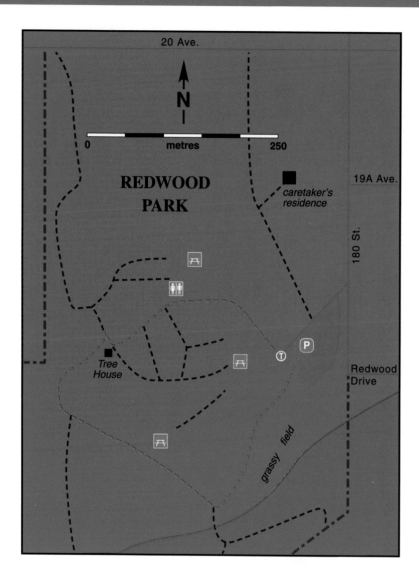

Find the paved path at the northwestern corner of the parking area and follow it past a playground area and past the washroom building. Where the path enters the forest, the pavement is replaced by gravel. Walk a few minutes more and you'll come to the Tree House.

Take the trail to the right of the Tree House. About 300 metres along the path, look on the left for a dirt trail. Go left. A short walk along this dirt trail brings you to the base of a big, reddish-brown tree (see p. 174).

Continue beyond the sequoia to follow the trail beneath some western redcedar trees and past some foamflowers. As you walk along, be sure to look for dead trees. When you see a snag, see if you can spot one of its regular visitors—a pileated woodpecker (see p. 175). Listen and look. You might hear the familiar *rat-a-tat-tat* of a woodpecker at work, or you might see a small pile of chipped wood at the base of the snag.

Continue downhill and past a toppled tree. You soon come to a fork in the trail. Go left to a T junction where there is a rock. Continue straight ahead as the forest changes from mostly coniferous to mostly deciduous. If you're here in summer, there should be lots of wildflowers along the trail, including pink herb-Robert and yellow creeping buttercup (see p. 175).

The trail soon leads you to an open grassy area. The parking area is just ahead to the left.

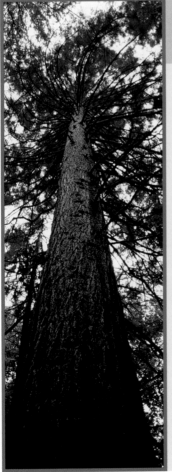

Giant Sequoia (*Sequoiadendron giganteum*)

Also known as the Sierra redwood, this species of tree is the one from which the park takes its name. Native to California, it does not grow in the wild in BC.

The giant sequoia can grow as tall as many downtown office buildings. The largest giant sequoia of all, the General Sherman tree located in California's Sequoia National Park, is 82.5 metres tall and more than 28 metres around. Although BC has taller trees (one Sitka spruce on Vancouver Island stands 96 metres tall) they're not as big around (the same spruce is only about 9.5 metres around). The General Sherman tree is not only considered to be the largest tree on earth, it's also considered to be the largest single living organism on earth.

Sequoias can also live to be very old. The General Sherman tree is believed to be about 2500 years old. The oldest giant sequoia that has been dated was more than 3200 years old when it was cut down.

The giant sequoias here in Redwood Park are just babies by comparison.

Pileated Woodpecker (Dryocopus pileatus)

The pileated woodpecker is the biggest woodpecker found in BC. About the same size as a crow, it's easy to recognize by the crest of bright red feathers on top of its head. Both the male and female have bright red crests, but only the male has bright red cheek feathers that look like a red moustache.

The pileated woodpecker eats mostly insects, although it will also eat berries

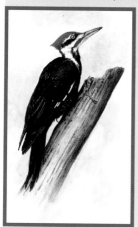

if they're around. To get at insects, it uses its sharp bill to hammer and chisel into the wood, usually a snag. Then it uses its long tongue to retrieve the bugs or grubs. Woodpeckers have thick, spongy skulls that absorb the shock of all that hammering, and their bills constantly grow, to replace what has worn away at the tip.

If you see a pileated woodpecker, notice how it holds onto the snag. Unlike most birds, which have three toes pointing forward and one backward, the pileated woodpecker has two toes pointing forward and two backward. This arrangement helps the bird hang on better. It also uses its tailfeathers to steady itself against the tree.

Creeping Buttercup (Ranunculus repens)

The creeping buttercup is not native to BC; it was introduced from Europe. It's considered a pest in some places because it can spread quickly through gardens and lawns, pushing out other flowers.

Some members of the buttercup family produce a substance in their leaves that can be poisonous, so most animals avoid eating buttercups. If a cow or a horse grazing in a field with buttercups in it accidentally eats some, the substance will irritate its mouth and digestive tract. If the buttercup is dried, it loses its toxicity and won't harm the animals.

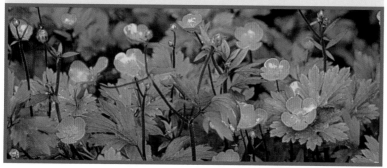

Tynehead Regional Park

Length: 2.5-km loop

Time needed: 1.5 to 2 hours

Season: Year-round

Rating: Easy; mostly flat terrain with a couple of short uphills

Dogs: Yes, on leash

Stroller-friendly: All-terrain stroller only

Washrooms: Outhouses at Serpentine Hollow picnic area

Highlights: Butterfly garden, big stumps, Serpentine River

Access: Follow Highway 1 (Upper Levels Highway) eastbound to Surrey and take exit 50 (160th Street and 104th Avenue). At 160th Street, go right. About 50 metres farther, turn left onto 103rd Avenue. Follow the green and yellow signs southward on 161st Street to the Serpentine Hollow picnic area parking lot.

Driving time: 40 minutes

The trails of Tynehead Regional Park are only minutes from the Trans-Canada Highway, but you'd never know it. Here, among the trees and along the river, is a peaceful place to wander. On a hot summer day it's a refreshingly cool and shady outing.

Take the trail on the left side of the parking area signboard. Walk past thimbleberries, old stumps, seedling trees and bigleaf maples. You will come to a boardwalk section that leads to a picnic area. Follow the trail to the right. After just a few steps on the next section of boardwalk, you'll find yourself in front of a butterfly garden.

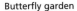
Butterfly garden

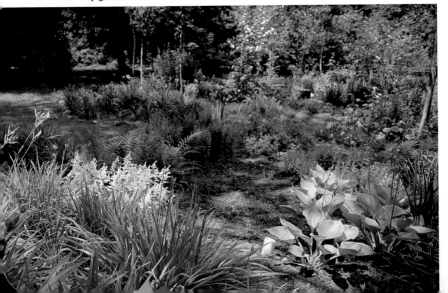

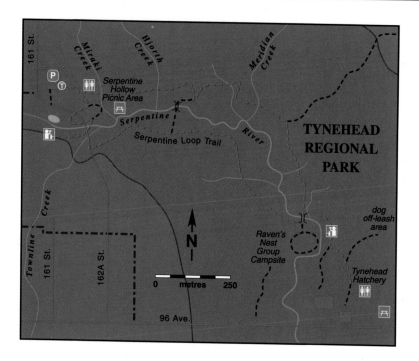

The Butterfly Garden

A butterfly garden has been created by planting the kinds of flowers and shrubs that butterflies like. Some of the flowers provide nectar for the butterflies. Other plants provide food for butterflies-in-waiting, also known as caterpillars.

Among the nectar plants are clover, buddleia (also called butterfly bush), dandelion, lilac, daisies and thistles. Among the food plants for caterpillars are willows, stinging nettle, spiraea and alder.

Some of the butterflies that you might see here are yellow tiger swallowtails, spring azures and red admirals.

Follow the trail as it loops around to the bridge. Cross the bridge over the Serpentine River. To the right is an optional side trip to a viewpoint that overlooks Serpentine Hollow. It's a short, steep climb, but the different perspective you get of the mixed forest is worth the effort and the 10 to 15 minutes it'll take to both go up and come back. There's also a western hemlock that's growing right through the viewing platform.

Once you're back down, cross the bridge over Townline Creek, and, where the trail forks, go left. You pass salmonberry and thimbleberry bushes, then you come to what looks like a toppled tree (see p. 178).

As you continue along the trail into the forest, notice the sapsucker holes on a big western hemlock on the left and more big nurse stumps on the right. The trail meanders through the forest of mixed deciduous and coniferous trees for 10 minutes or so and you soon come to a junction.

Keep right and go toward the Tynehead Hatchery. (Left takes you back over the Serpentine River, where you'd then meet up with the Sunny Trail, which returns to the parking area, for a short round trip of about 30 minutes.) The trail continues through lush forest where you might hear the chatter of Douglas's squirrels or the spiralling song of a Swainson's thrush.

A few minutes later, the trail forks. Go left. (Right leads to an open meadow.) A few minutes, at the next trail junction, go left onto a bridge over the Serpentine River.

Once you're across the bridge, you'll need to make a decision. You can go right for a quick side trip to the Tynehead Hatchery. (Tours can be arranged by appointment. Call (604) 589-9127 and leave a message.) Or you can go left. The trail passes through forest, then open meadow, then forest again, then open meadow again.

A few minutes along you'll pass the junction with the trail leading to the 168th Street entrance, then across a bridge over a small creek.

The Toppled Nurse Stump

At first glance, what you are looking at appears to be a single tree that might have been blown down by some big wind. But, if you look closer, you'll see that it's actually a cluster of western hemlock trees that grew on top of an old nurse stump. What likely happened is that, as the trees grew, their combined weight became too much for the decaying roots of the old nurse stump and so they all fell over. You can see the shallower old roots of the stump entwined with the newer, deeper roots of the hemlocks.

If you look even more closely, you can see all sorts of interesting clues to what's happened to both the old tree and the new ones. There are rusting nails

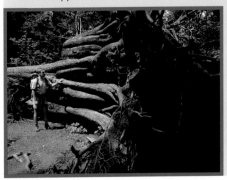

and a springboard hole on the stump from when the tree was logged. (The area was first logged in the 1880s.) There are squarish holes drilled in the stump's side where woodpeckers searched for insects. And on the trunks of the western hemlocks, there are neat rows of holes drilled by sapsuckers.

The trail will then wander through a section of forest that is mostly red alder. This is a great place to see and hear some of the birds that live in Tynehead, including the black-capped chickadee.

Continue along the trail, crossing the bridge over Meridian Creek. A bit farther is a big stump that's hollow inside. You can walk right in and check out the charred wood and the unburned parts where animals and birds have searched for insects. The trail continues past more big stumps then crosses another bridge.

You will soon come to a trail junction. Go right, then left and follow the signs toward the Serpentine Hollow picnic area. Cross the bridge over Hjorth Creek and look on the left of the trail for a really big Sitka spruce tree. You will then cross the bridge over Miraki Creek.

At the top of the stairs is a trail junction. Go right to return to the parking area.

Fish in the Serpentine River

The Serpentine River starts just west of this bridge, then runs about 27 kilometres to empty into the sea at Mud Bay. (See Serpentine Fen, p. 164.) Lots of little creeks and streams empty into the river along the way. That's both a good thing and a not-so-good thing. Because all the creeks and streams run through area that has been developed—as farms, housing or industrial areas—the water picks up pollution along the way.

It's especially bad news for the fish that live here—coho, chinook and chum salmon, and steelhead, cutthroat and rainbow trout. That's part of the reason a hatchery has been set up here at the park. Each year, the Tynehead Hatchery raises about 250,000 salmon and trout eggs until they are small fish called fry. Then the fry are released into the river and swim their way to the sea. They live in the sea for a number of years, then return to the river to spawn.

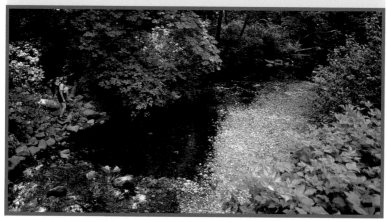

Campbell Valley

Length: 4-km loop

Time needed: 2 to 2.5 hours

Season: Year-round

Rating: Easy

Dogs: Yes, on leash

Stroller-friendly: All-terrain stroller only

Washrooms: At South Valley trailhead and at North Valley (halfway point)

Highlights: Bullfrogs, maples, Little Campbell River, squirrels

Access: Take Highway 99 south to exit 2 (Langley 8th Avenue East). Continue on 8th Avenue (Campbell River Road) east for about 7.5 kilometres, following the green and yellow signs to Campbell Valley Regional Park. Just past 200th Street is the South Valley entrance.

Driving time: 1 hour

Tucked away in Langley, near the US/Canada border, is a gem of a regional park. It's well known by horse riders for its equestrian trails. But there are also hiking trails that wander through forest, meadow and riverside groves.

From the parking area, head first toward the Visitor Centre and demonstration wildlife garden. If you're here between the middle of June and the end of August, you can tour the centre and check out their hands-on displays. Then take a stroll through the garden to see what species of trees, shrubs and flowers have been planted to attract wildlife—especially butterflies.

Take a short stroll to the ponds just north of the Visitor Centre. Rabbits run here and there over the grounds. And in the water, among all the vegetation, there are some very big frogs.

Bullfrog pond, Campbell Valley

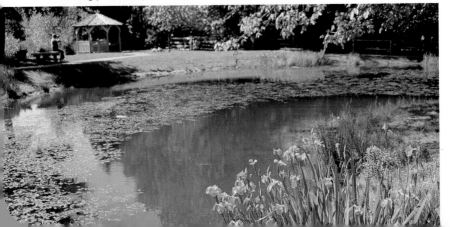

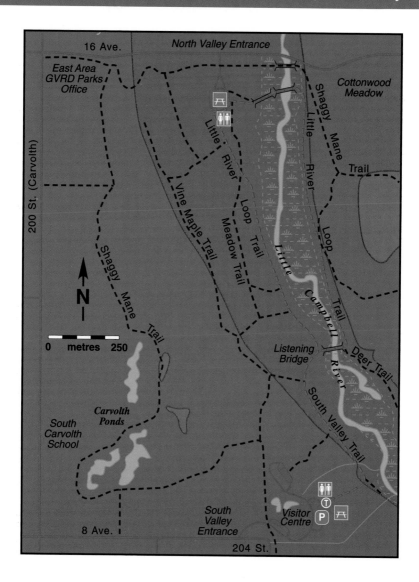

Bullfrogs

Bullfrogs are the biggest frogs found in BC. But they're not supposed to be here. They were introduced around the 1920s to be raised for frog's legs. Some frogs got loose, and it was bad news for the smaller frogs native to BC. These smaller frogs, such as the red-legged frog and the spotted frog, can't compete with the bigger bullfrog for food or habitat. Also, bullfrogs sometimes eat smaller frogs. Bullfrogs also eat turtle hatchlings, ducklings and certain birds.

Now, follow the trail just to the right of the Old Orchard picnic area sign, past the washrooms to the picnic area. At the trail junction, go left to follow the sign 'North Valley (16th Avenue) Entrance 1.3 kilometres.' The trail leads down through a lush deciduous forest of bigleaf maple and red alder.

In about 15 minutes, you'll come to another junction. Go right and soon you'll be on the Listening Bridge. Interpretive signs tell you more about the waterway that runs just below.

At the end of the bridge, go left and wander through more cool green forest. Walk for about 15 minutes to reach a huge bigleaf maple tree. On the other side of the path is a vine maple. Take a moment to look at the differences between these two native maple trees.

Continue north and follow the trail as it curves west and crosses two more bridges over the Little Campbell River. Where the trail forks, go left. You soon arrive at the north parking lot. Just past the washrooms is the continuation of the Little River Loop Trail.

Go left and continue your rambling through more open forest. You'll likely hear plenty of bird songs here as well as the chattering and scolding of another forest resident: Douglas's squirrel (see p. 183).

Soon, the trail leads back past the junction to the Listening Bridge. Keep going back up the South Valley Trail back to the picnic area and a little farther to the parking lot.

Bigleaf Maple (Acer macrophyllum) & Vine Maple (Acer circinatum)

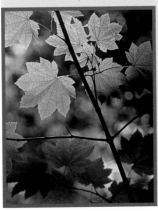

Bigleaf maples (up to 35 metres tall) are bigger than vine maples, which grow to only about 7 metres tall. As well, bigleaf maples have bigger leaves than vine maples do. A closer look at the leaves shows more differences— bigleaf maple leaves have five lobes, or points, and vine maple leaves (shown in photo) have either seven or nine lobes. The autumn leaves are also different colours— vine maple leaves turn red, and bigleaf maple leaves turn yellow.

These two trees may be quite different, but they do belong to the same genus, or group, of trees—Acer. They both like to grow in moist places and they both have seed pods, called samaras, that look like wings. If you throw samaras up in the air, they come twirling down like little helicopters.

Little Campbell River

The Little Campbell River doesn't look much like a river. In fact, in summer, it can be hard to see the calm brownish water at all because of all the marsh plants that grow here.

Although it may not look like much, the Little Campbell River is very important habitat for many different species of plants and animals. Take fish, for example. Beneath the water's surface are black crappies and three-spine sticklebacks as well as very young chum, coho and chinook salmon, called fry. They thrive in places like this where there's lots of food—mostly insects and insect larvae—and few predators.

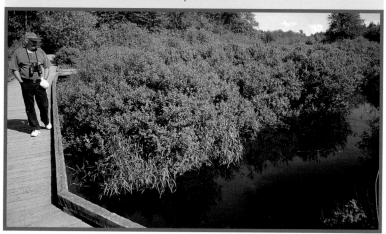

Douglas's Squirrel *(Tamiasciurus douglasi)*

These squirrels, unlike the grey squirrels you might have seen in Stanley Park, are native to BC. They're usually light brown, with a somewhat paler belly. And in winter, their ears have little pointy tufts of brown fur.

They eat mostly seeds, berries, nuts and mushrooms. Some of their favourite seeds come from Douglas-fir cones and bigleaf maple samaras.

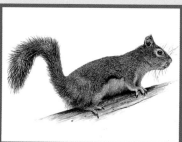

Squirrels build nests in dead trees, using strips of cedar bark and moss. Once a year, they have a litter of four to eight babies.

Douglas's squirrels can live up to seven years in the wild. Most don't make it past three years because of all the other animals—such as hawks, bobcats and weasels—that eat them.

Derby Reach

Length: 5-km loop

Time needed: 2 to 2.5 hours

Season: Year-round

Rating: Moderate

Dogs: Yes, on leash

Stroller-friendly: All-terrain stroller only

Washrooms: At trailhead

Highlights: Fraser River, Oregon grape, licorice fern, heritage buildings

Access: Take Highway 1 (Upper Levels Highway) to Langley. Take the 200th Street exit (#58) and head north to 88th Avenue. Go right on 88th to 208th Street, then turn left and follow it to Allard Crescent. Go right and follow the green and yellow GVRD signs for 4.3 kilometres to the Houston Trailhead.

Driving time: 1 hour

Derby Reach Regional Park is a bit of an undiscovered treasure. Although people who live in Langley are regular visitors, many other people have never even heard of the park, let alone visited it.

If you go, you'll be pleasantly surprised. Our hike starts with views of the Fraser River and the mountains beyond, then continues past a beaver dam and along a rolling trail through rainforest that is green even in the dead of winter.

Derby Reach trail

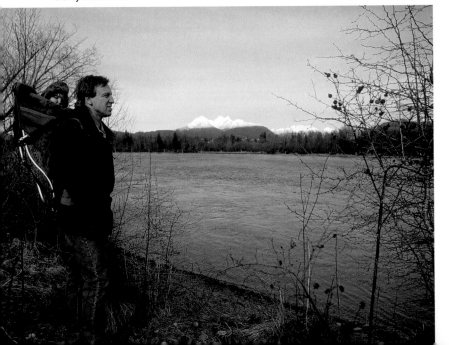

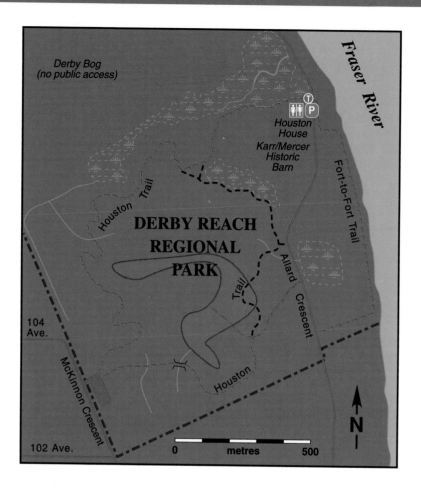

Once you've parked in the lot, cross the street to the Fort-to-Fort Trail and go right. This wide gravel path is just part of a much longer trail that will eventually connect Fort Langley to this place, called Derby Townsite, where the very first Fort Langley once stood.

As the trail heads south along the Fraser River, it crosses an open meadow area—a good place to see birds almost any time of year. In summer, there are lots of songbirds that flit and feed among the grasses. And in winter, there always seem to be a lot of robins that hang out here.

The trail heads up a little hill and then comes to a wooden platform and viewpoint. In the distance are mountains such as Golden Ears, Alouette and Robie Reid. If you look downriver, you might also see Mount Baker. Then take a look at the river in front of you.

As the trail continues, it passes some farmhouses and a small pond on the right. In winter, ducks can be seen paddling and dabbling.

Soon, the trail heads back toward the road. Cross the road and go right (so that you're walking against traffic). You'll pass another small pond on the left where you can see ducks and evidence of beavers. You might notice the chickenwire that has been wrapped around tree bottoms to keep the beavers from chewing them down. Or you might notice the long row of chewed-off branches and twigs where the pond comes to an end. (You probably won't see the beavers, though. They're pretty shy animals and tend to come out only early in the morning and around sunset.)

When you come to the yellow gate, go left and uphill. There's a great big cottonwood tree on the right. You can recognize it by the bark on its trunk—it looks like a freshly plowed field. In spring, summer and autumn, you can also look for the telltale heart-shaped leaves.

In winter, most of the trees here are leafless. But there is still a lot of green to be seen with all the moss, ferns and other shrubs growing on the forest floor. One of the shrubs you can look for is called Oregon grape (see p. 187). As you near the top of the hill, look on the right side for its big bunches of shiny, green, holly-like leaves.

Not much farther is a trail junction. Go left. If you want only a short walk of about one hour, you can go right and return to the heritage area and the parking lot.

The Fraser River

The Fraser River is the longest river in BC. It starts near Mount Robson in the Rocky Mountains and travels almost 1380 kilometres to reach the Pacific Ocean.

The Fraser is also the largest salmon-producing river in the world. About 800 million juvenile salmon migrate down the Fraser each year. And each of those salmon can spend up to three months in the estuary part of the Fraser—the part in the Lower Mainland—feeding and adjusting to salt water, before heading out to sea.

You likely won't see any salmon from this trail, but you may see boats that fish for salmon. And you might see other things that are affecting the numbers and the health of the salmon in the river—such things as urban growth, sewage and pollution.

In 2001, the Outdoor Recreation Council of BC named the Fraser the number four endangered river in BC. In a way, that's actually a bit of good news—it used to be the number one endangered river in the province. And although certain things have been done to make the river cleaner and healthier, much work still remains. For example, damaged habitat for fish and wildlife needs to be restored, water quality needs to be improved and gravel needs to be removed.

Oregon Grape *(Mahonia nervosa)*

Oregon grape is native to southwestern BC. In spring, it has bright yellow flowers. And later in summer it will have purply blue berries. They look a bit like small grapes, but they don't taste like grapes.

The berries are edible but can taste pretty sour. The First Nations people of southwestern BC used to collect the berries for eating. Some were eaten right off the bush, and others were mixed with huckleberries and/or salal berries, then boiled, mashed and dried into cakes.

It's also possible to make jelly or wine from Oregon grapes. But don't take too many berries, because many birds depend on them for food.

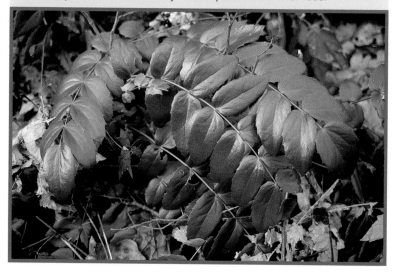

The forest now is mostly red alder and vine maple, much of it wrapped in layers of moss and lichen. There are a few western redcedars. And you might also hear Pacific tree frogs, whose singing and chirping sound almost like birds.

About 15 to 20 minutes of walking will bring you to the trailhead at McKinnon Crescent. Take a look at the map on the signboard just to see where you are and where you are going, then head right and follow the path as it returns back to the forest.

There are more trees covered with moss, moss and more moss. But you might also notice a certain kind of fern growing from the trunks of these trees. It's called licorice fern (see p. 188).

As the trail continues, the forest changes a bit. There are fewer deciduous trees, such as alders and maples. But there are more coniferous trees, such as western hemlock, Douglas-fir and Sitka spruce.

Licorice Fern *(Polypodium glycyrrhiza)*

Licorice ferns are often found growing on bigleaf maple tree trunks, but they also grow on logs, rocks and wet, mossy ground. This fern's whitish rhizome, a kind of root-like stem, tastes like licorice, which explains the name.

The rhizomes were chewed by some First Nations peoples for colds or sore throats. Other First Nations peoples used them as a sweetener for food or medicine. And others just chewed on them for a bit of flavour.

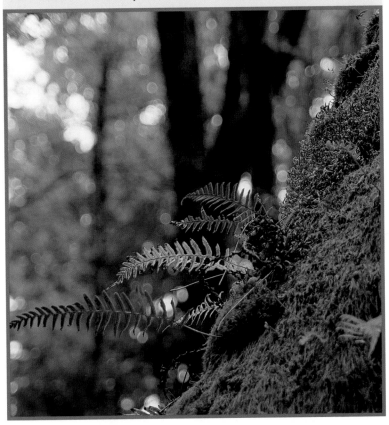

About 30 minutes from the McKinnon Crescent trailhead, the trail forks. Go left toward the heritage area. The trail passes through an open meadow then emerges to views of a large marsh and distant mountains. (Do they look familiar? They're the same ones you saw at the start of the hike.)

You will soon return to the heritage area. Go right through the fence to return to the parking lot. But first, take a moment to check out some of the old buildings.

Heritage Buildings

People have lived at Derby Reach for a long time. Although the First Nations people were the first to inhabit the area, the buildings they lived in are no longer around.

That's also the case with buildings from the first Fort Langley, which was built here in 1827 and later relocated to the place it is now—a few kilometres up-river. There are also no buildings left from the original Derby townsite, established in 1858. On the main street, there was a hardware store, restaurants, a billiards hall, hotels, a bank and post office, a court house, church and jail. But by 1866, most of the people had left for other towns in the Lower Mainland, such as Fort Langley and New Westminster (then called Queensborough).

The buildings that stand here today date from the early 1900s. The house, which is currently rented out to caretakers, was built in 1908. The small building with the roof that looks a little too long is a milkhouse that was built in 1935 when all this area was the Houston Farm.

Then there's the great big barn just beyond. It's not the original barn that was here—it was too dilapidated to be restored. Instead this barn was built in 1876 in Rosedale (near Chilliwack) and moved here in 1989.

Heritage milkhouse

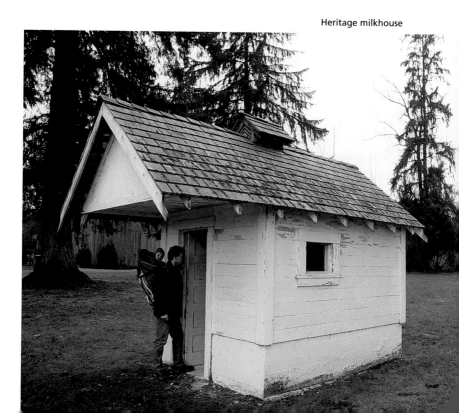

Burnaby Lake

Length: 5-km loop

Time needed: 2 to 2.5 hours

Season: Year-round

Rating: Easy

Dogs: Yes, on leash

Stroller-friendly: All-terrain stroller only

Washrooms: Behind the Nature House at Piper Spit

Highlights: Cariboo Dam, Brunette River, Sitka spruce, Piper Spit birds, spittlebugs

Access: Take Highway 1 (Upper Levels Highway) to the Gaglardi Way/Cariboo Road exit and follow Cariboo Road north to Avalon Avenue. Then turn left and follow the signs to the parking lot area.

Driving time: 30 minutes

You might not expect to find a wildlife haven squished between a major highway and an industrial area, but that's where you'll find the natural wonders of Burnaby Lake. The 300-hectare regional park is home to beavers, blackbirds, bugs and all kinds of other animals and plants. And there are lots of paths along the lakeshore to help you explore it all.

Starting from the parking area, look for and follow the signs toward Piper Spit. Very soon, you'll cross a cement dam (see below).

After crossing the dam, go left to follow the Brunette Headwaters Trail. If you go in summer, you'll see pink pond-lilies on the lake and white daisies on the lakeshore. About 10 to 15 minutes later, cross a wooden bridge over Silver Creek, one of many little creeks that bring water into Burnaby Lake.

A few minutes later, where two big trees straddle the trail, is an intersection. Go right to follow the Spruce Loop Trail. On the forest floor are lots of different plants: bracken fern, salmonberry and skunk cabbage, to name a few. You might also hear the rumble of a passing freight train. (The tracks are just on the other side of the trees.)

Where you cross a small wooden bridge, look for water striders, water boatmen and tiny fish in the tiny trickle of a creek. After 20 minutes or

The Cariboo Dam & the Brunette River

The Cariboo dam, like all dams, is here to help control water. It can help control how much water is in Burnaby Lake and how much water flows out of the lake and into the Brunette River.

The amounts of water in both the lake and the river are important. The lake needs to be a certain depth to be able to provide homes and food for fish and other wildlife. If too much water leaves the lake—such as might happen when it rains heavily—there could be flooding downstream.

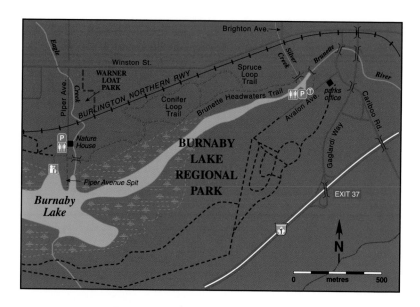

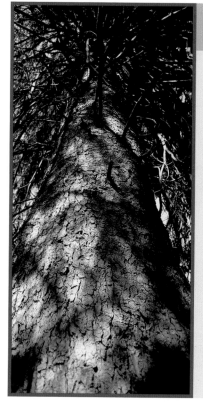

Sitka Spruce
(Picea sitchensis)

One of the easiest ways to identify a Sitka spruce is by its bark. It's greyish and scaly. If the needles are close enough, have a touch—but be careful. Sitka spruce needles are sharp. Look on the ground for cones. Sitka spruce cones are long—about as long as an adult's finger—and have overlapping scales.

This tree is big, but it's not as tall as some Sitka spruce trees that grow on Vancouver Island in Carmanah Pacific Provincial Park. Those trees stand around 90 metres high, about the same as some downtown office buildings or 45 adults standing one on top of the other.

The native peoples of BC used all parts of these trees—needles, bark, pitch, roots and branches—for many different purposes, including food, medicine and hats.

so, you'll join up with the Brunette Headwaters Trail again. Go right. Immediately on the left side of the trail is a big Sitka spruce.

Continue along the Brunette Headwaters Trail for another 10 to 15 minutes to the intersection with the Nature House pathway. Go right to visit the Nature House. It's open on weekends and statutory holidays from mid-May to Labour Day. There are lots of neat hands-on displays that can show you more about the plants and animals that live in and around Burnaby Lake.

After checking out the Nature House, amble back along the path toward the lake. This is one of the best places in the park to see birds. If you follow the Cottonwood Trail west for a few metres, you can climb up the viewing tower. From here, you can see from one end of the lake to the other. You can also see songbirds such as red-winged blackbirds, black-capped chickadees and barn swallows.

Piper Spit Birds

Most of the birds that you see here are ducks and geese. If you come here in winter, you'll see different kinds of ducks than you'd see during the rest of the year. That's because some ducks overwinter here where it's warmer and then fly north for the summer. That's where they'll lay eggs and raise their baby ducks. Then, in autumn, when it starts getting colder and snow begins to fall, they'll head south again to places where it's warmer and easier to get food.

A lot of people feed the ducks and geese here. If you want to feed them, make sure you give them birdseed, not bread. Because the grain in bread has been ground up, mixed and cooked, birds don't get any nutrition from it.

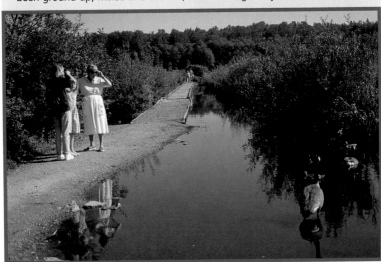

Spittlebugs (Order Homoptera)

When they are young and called nymphs, spittlebugs nestle into the space between a leaf and the stem. Then they ooze a froth of bubbles to protect themselves from dry air, predators and parasites. Concealed in their slimy nests, spittlebugs can feed on the plant juices. The nymphs are tiny—about the same size as a sesame seed. When they grow to adult size, spittlebugs are brown, with wings, and about the same size as a pea. They hop around a lot, which is why some people call them froghoppers.

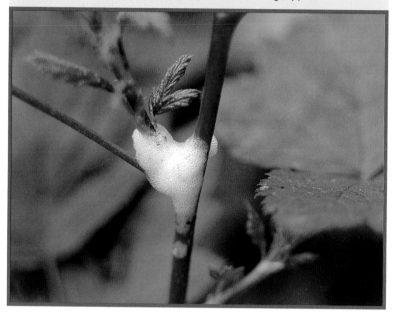

After climbing down, return to the intersection and head down along the skinny finger of land that pokes out into the water. It's called Piper Spit, and you can see even more birds here.

Once you've explored Piper Spit, just turn around and head back to Cariboo Dam. Cross the bridge over Eagle Creek and retrace your steps along the Brunette Headwaters Trail. When you come to trail intersections, stay straight ahead on the same trail rather than retracing the loop trails you did on the way in.

If you're here in spring or in summer, take a closer look at the plants around you. Do some leaves have a bunch of bubbles that look like someone spit on them? Well, in fact, 'someone' did—an insect called a spittlebug.

You soon reach the Cariboo Dam. Then, just cross over and return to the parking area.

Burnaby Mountain

Length: 4 km

Time needed: 2 to 2.5 hours

Season: Year-round

Rating: Moderate; rolling terrain with a number of hills

Dogs: Yes, on leash

Stroller-friendly: All-terrain stroller only

Washrooms: At Burnaby Mountain Park

Highlights: Siberian miner's-lettuce, Swainson's thrush, wood-eating bugs, geology

Access: Take Lougheed Highway east to Gaglardi Way in Burnaby. Turn left (north) and follow Gaglardi toward Simon Fraser University. Turn left (west) on Burnaby Mountain Parkway. At Centennial Way turn right, and follow it north to the parking lot at the end.

Driving time: 30 minutes

The many kilometres of trails on the top and sides of Burnaby Mountain have been popular with hikers since the 1920s. Now, they've also become popular with mountain bikers. This hike follows one of the north-side trails, recently upgraded as part of the Trans Canada Trail.

From the parking lot, follow the paved path past Horizons restaurant and the rose garden to the chain-link fence. Go right and follow the gravel path uphill, past the playground to the end of the fence. The trail starts here.

Staying left, you'll pass a water reservoir and, a bit farther, you'll come to a trail junction. Go left to enter a mixed forest of coniferous and deciduous trees. Big snags can be seen alongside the trail, remnants of the original forest that was logged from the 1900s to the 1940s.

In summer, you'll also likely notice hundreds of little white flowers alongside the trail. Stop and take a closer look at this oddly named wildflower (see p. 195).

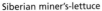

Siberian miner's-lettuce

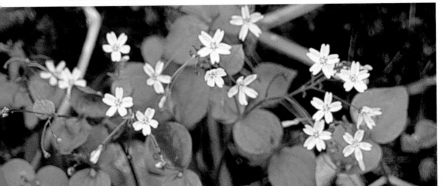

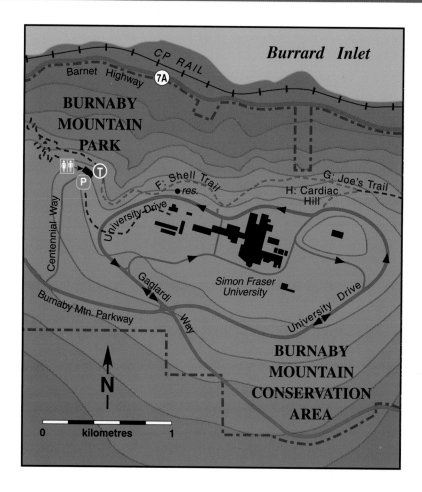

Siberian Miner's-lettuce *(Montia sibirica)*

Although the white or pink flowers of this plant may be pretty, the leaves and stem are pretty interesting, too. As the name suggests, they were eaten as salad greens (lettuce) by early prospectors or miners. Sometimes, the leaves and stems were cooked. They're said to taste like spinach.

The leaves are a source of vitamins A and C—precious nutrients to prospectors and miners without access to many vegetables, let alone super-markets and tropical produce.

BC's First Nations peoples didn't eat Siberian miner's-lettuce, but they did use the plant as a medicine to help ease such ailments as constipation and headaches.

Swainson's Thrush (*Catharus ustulatus*)

These starling-sized birds are hard to spot amid all the ferns, shrubs and trees. They're not colourful—shades of brown and grey—and they spend much of their time on the ground, foraging for insects, spiders and berries.

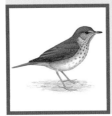

But you can't miss their song. It sounds like someone playing a flute, starting with one clear long note, then spiralling up the scale and fading out.

Swainson's thrushes aren't here year-round. They arrive sometime in May to build nests, lay eggs and raise their young. By October, they leave for their wintering grounds in Central America and South America.

The trail wanders past more snags and more living trees—western redcedars, western hemlocks and lots of red alder. You'll also see shrubs such as huckleberry, red elderberry and even some devil's club.

You may also see birds flitting here and there among all the foliage. But use your sense of hearing as well, and you'll detect woodpeckers, golden-crowned kinglets and winter wrens. Between May and October, you may also hear the unmistakable song of the Swainson's thrush.

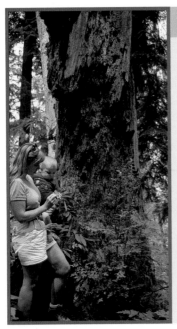

Wood-eaters

Ants, beetles and woodborers are just a few kinds of insects you might see here. They help chew up the wood and break it down into substances that plants can use for food, and in turn they themselves are food for birds, bears and other insect-eating animals.

Some insects have enzymes in their stomachs that can digest cellulose—the main component of wood—but others don't. They depend on the bacteria that live in their stomachs to break cellulose down. Other insects may eat the wood but only digest the fungi that are on the dead wood, also helping to break it down.

You may also see some other non-insect bugs such as sowbugs, millipedes and spiders.

The trail levels, then climbs gradually. Soon, there is a junction with the F trail. Stay left. You will cross a bridge over a ravine. Not much farther is a big snag on the left side of the trail. Take a close look at the deteriorating bark to see some of the insects that are burrowing in or slowly eating the remains of this dead tree.

Continue following the trail as it descends. Then, just when you hear the tinkling of a small creek, the upper side of the trail changes from shrub-covered slope to exposed layers of rock and silt (see below).

The trail descends a bit more, then passes a more open area of alder forest with the occasional view of Belcarra across the water and of the North Shore mountains in the distance. Continue a bit farther to a junction with trail H, also known as Cardiac Hill.

Now you must decide whether to return the same way you came, or, if you don't mind walking along a roadside, to go up Cardiac Hill—10 to 15 minutes of steep trail—and follow University Drive west for another 30 to 40 minutes. If you take the latter route, continue along the roadside past the service station to a stoplight. Then, follow the trail that veers away from the road and into the trees. It will lead you back to the parking area where you started.

Geological History

At one point, probably around 40 to 45 million years ago, Burnaby Mountain was part of a flat river plain that covered most of southwestern BC. You can see the layers of pebbles and small rocks that would have been brought here by rivers that flowed from the north. These layers are mixed with layers of silt and sand. About five million years ago, the whole Coast Mountain area was pushed upward by geological forces. Erosion by water, wind and ice sculpted Burnaby Mountain into the form it is today.

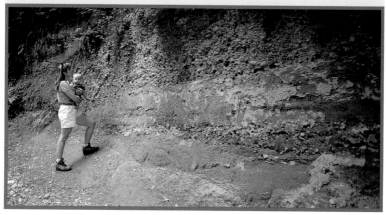

Fraser Foreshore

Length: 4.5 km

Time needed: 2 to 2.5 hours

Season: Year-round

Rating: Easy

Dogs: Yes, on leash

Stroller-friendly: Yes

Washrooms: In building near playground

Highlights: Paper birch, thimbleberry, Fraser River, sparrows

Access: Take SE Marine Drive east toward Burnaby. Just past Kerr Street, bear right to follow Marine Way until you reach Byrne Road. Go right and to the end of Byrne Road where you'll find Fraser Foreshore Park.

Driving time: 25 minutes

For a lovely walk along the Fraser River, complete with views, big cottonwood trees and lots of birdlife, Fraser Foreshore is the place to go. The trail is wide and well maintained. The park features a playground and picnic tables as well.

From the parking area, head west along the paved path past a pumphouse, where the path turns to gravel. Trees line both sides of the path. Most are black cottonwood trees with their familiar heart-shaped leaves. But look for one tree that's different from all the others—a paper birch tree. You'll find it just opposite the big stump.

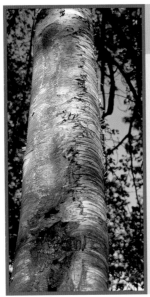

Paper Birch
(Betula papyrifera)

The easiest way to tell a paper birch from other trees is by its bark. It tends to peel off like strips of paper. Sometimes the bark is white, other times—as with this tree—it's more of a coppery brown.

Paper birch has been used by native peoples of North America for thousands of years. The bark was used to make baskets, cradles and canoes. But other parts of the tree found uses as well. The sap and the inner bark were used as food in times of famine. The leaves were used to make soap and shampoo.

It's important, though, that you don't try to strip any bark from the tree. That can cause big ugly scars and may even kill the tree.

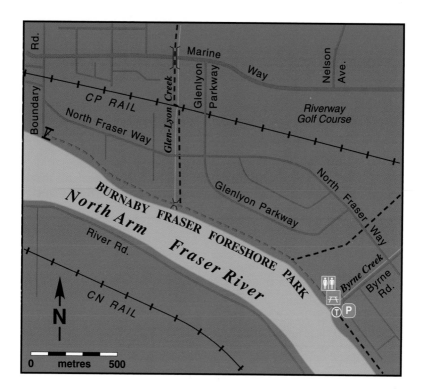

The trail continues, crossing Byrne Creek, then passes an open area
with views of Burnaby city and, farther in the distance, the North Shore
mountains. (You can even see The Lions.) Cross a wooden bridge and
you'll come to a fork in the path. Go left. You'll soon cross another bridge.
On the right is part of an industrial park, but continue along the riverside.

In spring and summer, the shrubs can be quite dense, allowing only the
occasional glimpse of the river. So, take a look at the shrubs themselves
and see how many different species you can see. Among them are wild
rose, twinberry and thimbleberry (see p. 200).

You will come to a sign showing the Fraser Foreshore trails and your
location on the trail. Continue straight ahead. Just beyond is an opening
with a good view of the Fraser River. This part of the river is called the
North Arm. That's because just a bit farther east, near New Westminster,
the Fraser splits into two parts—north and south—as it comes through
the Lower Mainland. The North Arm passes Burnaby, Vancouver and
Richmond on its way to the sea.

Continue along through more dense shrubs. In places like this, you'll
often see or hear birds. Sometimes you may hear rustling in the shrubs,
near the ground. Many people think these rustlings are made by garter

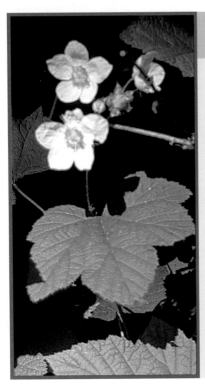

Thimbleberry
(Rubus parviflorus)

If you see a thimbleberry bush when it is in blossom, you might mistake it for a blackberry bush. But look a little closer. While both plants have white flowers, thimbleberry doesn't have the nasty sharp prickles that blackberry does. The white flowers are also a bit bigger and more delicate.

The berries are quite different, too. Blackberries are big, black and sweet. Thimbleberries look like rather flat raspberries and can taste bland.

Northwest coast First Nations peoples used to gather thimbleberries for food—often using the big soft thimbleberry leaves as containers. Sometimes they ate them fresh. Other times, they dried the berries and made them into cakes.

Sparrows

About 11 species of sparrow can be found in the Lower Mainland. Some, such as the chipping sparrow, are rarely seen. Others, such as song sparrows, can be seen almost anywhere there is suitable habitat.

Some sparrow species, such as the white-crowned sparrow (illustrated), are fairly easy to identify using a field guide. But others, known among birders as 'LBJs' or 'little brown jobs,' are difficult to tell apart.

All sparrows have cone-shaped bills. The shape is the perfect tool for sparrows' favourite food: seeds. (In summer, sparrows will also eat insects and fruit.) 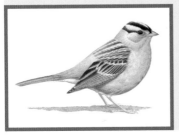 Some species of sparrow have developed techniques to help them find food on the ground. White-crowned and Lincoln's sparrows use their feet to scratch and uncover seed and bugs. The fox sparrow takes it one step further, often jumping back and forth, pulling aside dead leaves and brush to uncover food.

snakes or mice, but in fact, most of the time it's birds making the noise. Among the various birds you might see are sparrows (see p. 200).

The path soon emerges to another outfall pipe and another industrial park. The trail continues for another 5 to 10 minutes. On the right is industrial park; on the left is river. Finally, you come to the end—a gate and Boundary Road. There's also a gazebo and bench where you can take a short rest before retracing your steps to the parking area.

A Working River

The Fraser is often called a 'working river,' which means that people depend upon it for a lot of things related to work. On this part of the Fraser, you can see tugboats pulling barges, boats and other things, such as log booms.

Even in the early 1900s, people depended on the Fraser River. Loggers who cut trees in what is now Burnaby would float the logs down Byrne Creek and into the Fraser. Then they were floated to sawmills farther east in New Westminster.

These days, trees are no longer logged in Burnaby, but you can still see lots of logs tied up along the shore. Many of them are waiting to go to the MacMillan Bloedel mill that you can see just across from the end of the trail.

It's not just mills that have used the Fraser. Other industries set up business along the Fraser because it made transporting goods so easy. The only problem with working rivers is that they are often polluted by the industries that depend on them. If the rivers are damaged, so are the habitats of the fish and the other animals that live there.

People are working to restore the Fraser to a better state of health, but the problems will take much more time to fix than they did to create.

Fraser River

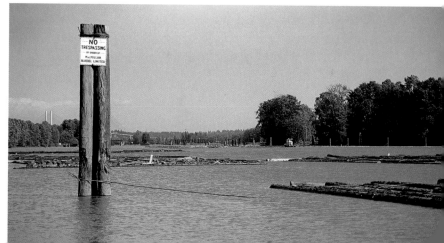

Shoreline Park

Length: 4 km

Time needed: 2 to 2.5 hours

Season: Year-round

Rating: Easy

Dogs: Yes, on leash

Stroller-friendly: All-terrain stroller only

Washrooms: At Rocky Point Park

Highlights: Old fish boat, salmonberry, Nootka rose, hatchery

Access: Take Barnet Highway to St. Johns Street in Port Moody. At Moody Street, turn left (north) and follow the overpass as it loops to the west. At the stop sign turn left onto Murray Street, and then left again into the parking area for Rocky Point Park.

Driving time: 35 minutes

Shoreline Park is the official name for a lovely trail that meanders around the eastern end of Burrard Inlet. You'll wander through shaded forest and over boardwalks on mud-flats and find interesting little side trails along the way.

Fish Packer

It's not known how this boat came to be here, but it's been here for as long as most people remember. Each year the wreck gets a bit smaller as pieces of wood break off and float away. Although people sometimes break the wood off and carry it away, much of the deterioration is from the water, mud and marine organisms that are slowly eroding the wood.

Some of the most obvious creatures that live on the wreck are barnacles. They don't actually eat the wood; they use it as an anchor. By sticking themselves to the wood—or metal—parts of the boat, they can push out their feathery 'hands' to catch plankton and other microscopic food floating by.

Just after high tide, you might also notice worm trails on the sand by the boat. These are left by thread worms—so named because they are very thin and long—that eat decaying plant matter, including old wood, in the water.

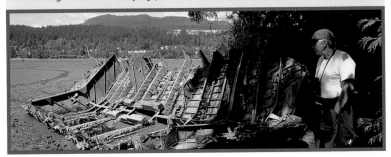

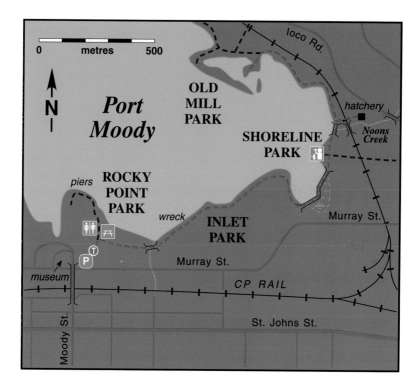

From the parking area, head right toward the playground. Then, follow the concrete path east until you cross a bridge. Go left on the gravel path. Scan the shoreline as you walk along, and soon, you'll see the dilapidated remains of an old boat. Short steep side trails lead down to the flats.

Back on the main trail, continue walking through a lovely forest of hemlock, cedar and vine maple trees. The understorey is made up of lots of plants and shrubs, including some—salal, huckleberry and salmonberry (see p. 204)—that dangle berries during the summer months.

As the trail continues, there are more bridges to cross and the occasional bench to sit on. At the next junction, about 15 minutes in, stay left along the shore. You will soon be walking on the boardwalk above the estuary of a tiny creek. In winter, it's mostly a mud-flat beneath the boardwalk. But in spring or summer, it'll look like you're walking through a field of grass.

On the other side of the boardwalk, the path is lined with wild rose bushes (see p. 204) and crabapple trees. A side trail goes left to a viewpoint with a bench. This is a great spot to have some lunch or a snack before continuing.

Back on the main trail, head in the same direction as earlier. Bigger alder and cottonwood trees now mix in with the smaller crabapple trees.

Salmonberry *(Rubus spectabilis)*

There are a couple of ways to tell the salmonberry shrubs from thimbleberry and huckleberry. If it's springtime, salmonberry shrubs have bright pink blossoms. If it's early summer, salmonberry shrubs have juicy berries that look like blackberries except they're yellow or red.

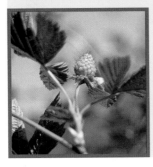

Salmonberries are very edible. Historically, they were eaten by all the First Nations peoples of the West Coast. Some would mix the berries with grease from a species of fish called an oolichan. Or the berries were eaten with salmon.

These days, salmonberries are still eaten by First Nations peoples, along with the new shoots of the salmonberry shrub. Sometimes, the shoots are peeled and eaten right away. Other times, the shoots are steamed.

A bit farther is more boardwalk. And then you come to Noons Creek. At the end of the boardwalk, look for a trail that breaks right. Follow it across the paved path to Noons Creek Hatchery. The Port Moody Ecological Society has operated the hatchery since 1991 and raises tiny chum and coho salmon and cutthroat trout that get released in the wild.

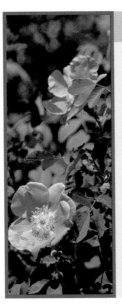

Nootka Rose *(Rosa nutkana)*

The Nootka rose is one of five different species of wild rose that grow in BC, and it is probably the most commonly seen wild rose in the Lower Mainland. These wild roses are different from the roses you buy at the store, but they do have some common features.

Both wild roses and cultivated roses have thorns. Both have leaves that look similar. And both smell wonderful.

In addition to having a nice smell, the Nootka rose also had other uses for First Nations peoples. It was used for food—its new shoots were eaten in spring. It was used in cooking food—its branches were used in steaming pits and cooking baskets. And it was used in making medicines—the bark, leaves, hips or fruit were used to help things such as sore eyes, bee stings and diarrhea.

Salmon Hatcheries

Streams and creeks, such as Noons Creek, used to have lots of salmon and trout living in them. But as people settled in the area, built houses and businesses, roads and railways, the streams, creeks and their fish suffered.

Now hatcheries, such as Noons Creek Hatchery, are trying to bring back the salmon. In autumn, as adult fish return to the creek, eggs are taken from the female, and milt, or fish sperm, is taken from the male. They're mixed together so the eggs are fertilized. Then the eggs are put in special trays and left to incubate. In spring, tiny salmon called alevins hatch. For the next few weeks, they feed from a large yolk sac under their belly.

Once the yolk sac is used up, the fish are called fry and they're moved to special troughs to be fed and raised until they're big enough to release into the creek. Fry can take up to a year to get ready to head for the sea. When they do, they're about 10 centimetres long and are called fingerlings. They remain at sea until maturity. Then they return to the creek where they were born.

To find out more about hatchery tours, call (604) 469-9106. But even if the hatchery is closed, it's still worth a look.

Retrace your steps to the boardwalk and continue to follow the shoreline trail to the right. A few minutes later is a bridge that crosses over a creek. Just beyond is the rusting hulk of a steam boiler from an old lumber mill. And a short ways away are the foundations of the old mill itself.

It's possible to continue along the trail for another kilometre or so to Old Orchard Park, but many families will want to turn around at this point. Just retrace your steps back to Rocky Point Park.

Noons Creek

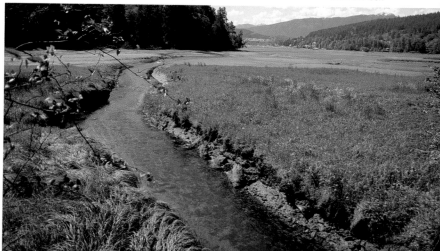

Admiralty Point

Length: 5 km

Time needed: 2 to 2.5 hours

Season: Year-round

Rating: Moderately easy; some uphill and uneven terrain

Dogs: Yes, on leash

Stroller-friendly: No

Washrooms: At parking area and at Maple Beach

Highlights: Shell middens, periwinkle, cabin remnants, Admiralty Point

Access: Take Barnet Highway to Port Moody. At Ioco Road, turn north and continue for about 4.5 kilometres to Sunnyside Road. Go right and follow the signs to the Belcarra Picnic Area along the recently built Tum-tumay-whueton Drive.

Driving time: 45 minutes

Located in Belcarra Regional Park, the Admiralty Point Trail offers a lovely seaside walk.

Before starting on the trail, first wander toward the beach. You're now standing on the site of what was once an important Coast Salish winter village called *Tum-tumay-whueton,* which means 'The Biggest Place for People.'

Ancient Inhabitants

Although you can't see them now, archaeologists have found shell middens—essentially ancient garbage dumps—here. In them were seeds, shells and bones from food that the Coast Salish people would have eaten. As well, the middens held other artifacts, such as broken and worn tools made from bone, antler and stone.

The middens date back to 1200 BC. The Tslaywuthuh band of the Salish Nation lived here during winter and spent summers in smaller camps farther up Indian Arm; in 1860, the band was relocated to the Burrard Reserve.

Cod Rock

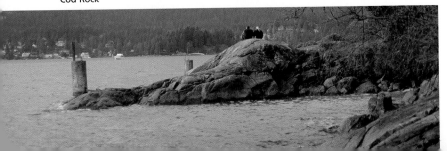

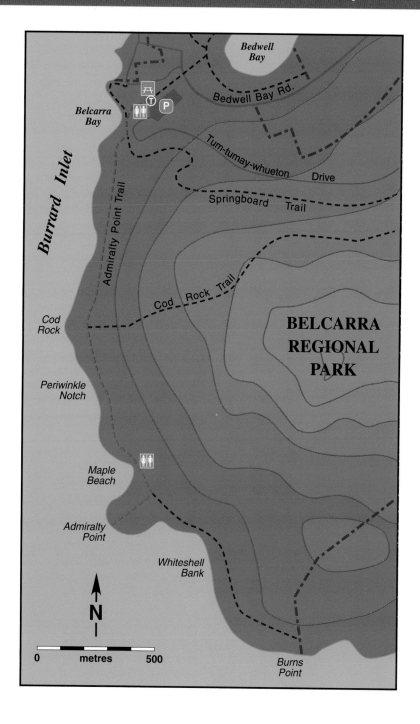

Bedwell
Bay

Bedwell Bay Rd.

Belcarra
Bay

Turn-tumay-whueton Drive

Admiralty Point Trail

Springboard Trail

Burrard Inlet

Cod Rock Trail

Cod
Rock

BELCARRA
REGIONAL
PARK

Periwinkle
Notch

Maple
Beach

Admiralty
Point

Whiteshell
Bank

N

0   metres   500

Burns
Point

Look for the start of the Admiralty Point Trail, located just behind the washroom building. A paved path leads to a wooden bridge over a small creek, and then becomes a gravel path that crosses a private road. Now comes the only real uphill part of the trail.

The trail climbs steadily through a mixed forest of deciduous and coniferous trees. In winter, when the alders and maples are bare of leaves, the trunks are clad in a green sweater of moss, lichen and fern.

Periwinkle (Vinca spp.)

The periwinkle flowers that grow here aren't native to BC but were planted by settlers. Throughout history, periwinkle has been used as medicine. In India, juice from the leaves was used to treat wasp stings. In Central and South America, people made a cough medicine from it. And in Hawaii, it was boiled to make a poultice (a kind of bandage). In Europe, people even thought the periwinkle was magic and could ward off evil spirits.

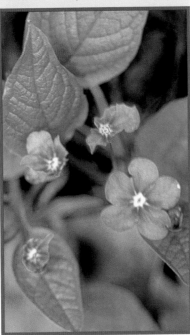

Not much farther, the trail passes rock outcrops dripping with moss, ferns, salal and other moisture-loving plants. Go a bit farther, then look on the right for an unmarked side trail that leads to Cod Rock.

From here, there are views north to Boulder Island and, farther beyond, North Vancouver and Mount Seymour. To the west is the Shellburn oil refinery and to the south is Burnaby Mountain.

Back on the main trail, pass a tiny stream and an old charred snag that gives some idea of how big the trees here once stood. A few steps farther, on the other side of the trail, is a stump with springboard holes that look like eyes. They date from the early 1900s when the area was logged. Now almost all the trees here are second-growth.

Cross another three small creeks and, just beyond a wooden fence, take the side trail to a rock outcrop at Periwinkle Notch—named for the periwinkle flowers found here.

Back on the trail, you might notice other things, such as old brick foundations and stone staircases (see p. 209). The trail leads past a few good-sized Douglas-fir trees, some with black bark from an ancient fire.

Cabin Remnants

Starting in the early 1900s, Belcarra was a popular place for people to come for their summer holidays. In 1923, the Harbour Navigation Company built a dance pavilion and 10 one-room cabins and planted an orchard.

On Fridays, a ferry would bring visitors from the city to Belcarra where they could picnic or stay in cabins for the weekend. This went on until about 1970 when the ferry service ended and the cabins were torn down.

However, even though they didn't own the land, people built 16 new cabins here and made themselves at home. But by 1982, when the GVRD began building the Admiralty Point Trail, many of the cabins had already been abandoned. The rest were dismantled as the trail was built.

The trail soon descends to Maple Beach, named for the cluster of bigleaf maples here. You'll probably notice the 'Bear in Area' sign. It's true, despite being so close to the city, you are in a wildlife area and could come across black bears, deer or even cougars.

Continue along the trail a bit farther, then take the side trail right to Admiralty Point (see below). When you've rested, maybe had some lunch or a snack, just retrace your steps to the Belcarra Picnic Area.

Admiralty Point

This point is named Admiralty Point. The tall ships that explored and traded along the West Coast came here during the 1800s and 1900s to find trees that were tall enough to be used as the main spars for the ships.

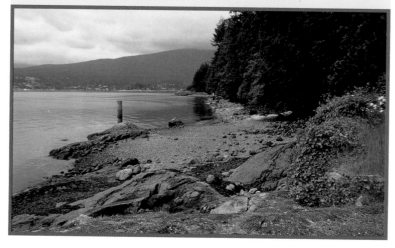

Mundy Lake

Length: 5-km loop

Time needed: 2 to 2.5 hours

Season: Year-round

Rating: Easy; one uphill section

Dogs: Yes, on leash

Stroller-friendly: All-terrain stroller only

Washrooms: On entrance road near parking area

Highlights: Lakes, water boatmen, yellow wood violets, snags

Access: Follow Lougheed Highway east to Austin Road. Go left and follow Austin for about 5 kilometres to Hillcrest Street. Turn left. Just past the playing field parking lot, look for a driveway on the right. Turn in and follow the road to the main parking area.

Driving time: 40 minutes

Mundy Park is one of Coquitlam's best-kept secrets. This 180-hectare park has more than 12 kilometres of trails that wander through second-growth forest and along lakesides. The forest is a haven of tranquillity lush with wildflowers, shrubs and birdsong.

From the parking area, head for the signboard and map. Go straight ahead, past the playing field and into the forest. Cross a bridge over Mundy Creek and at the first fork in the trail, go left. The trail then re-crosses Mundy Creek.

About 100 metres farther, look for the signpost pointing the way to Mundy Lake. Go right and soon you'll be on the shores of Mundy Lake.

Go left on the boardwalk as it skirts the shores of the lake. Farther on, there are a couple of opportunities to get closer to the water—and some of the lake's inhabitants.

Water Boatmen (Family Corixidae)

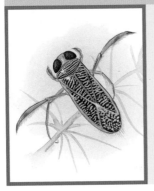

These little guys look a little different than the water striders almost everyone recognizes. Water striders skate across the water surface with their long skinny legs, whereas water boatmen look like they're rowing across the water.

The water boatman has three pairs of legs. The front legs are very short, and the water boatman uses them to collect algae and other tiny pieces of food. The middle legs are longer and used to hold onto plants. The back legs are the boatman's oars.

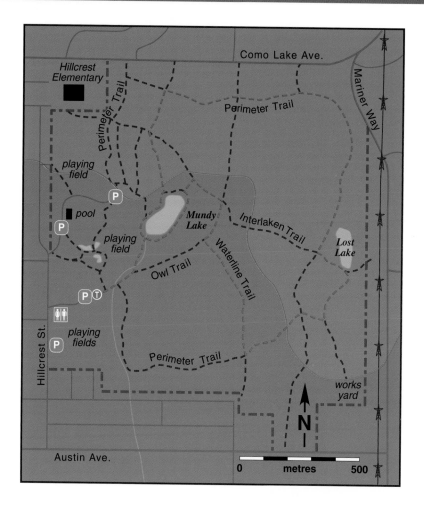

As you near the north end of the lake, look for a trail bearing left. Go left to follow the trail away from the lake and uphill via some long shallow steps. A short distance farther is a junction with the Interlaken Trail (also called the Orange Trail). Stay to the left for now.

At the next junction, go right to head east along the Perimeter Trail (also called the Blue Trail). Most of the trees here are less than 100 years old. The original forest was cut in the late 1890s, and you can still see the occasional stump or snag of those old-growth trees.

At the next junction, go right to continue on the Perimeter Trail. Here, you'll reach the highpoint of the hike, then the trail heads downhill. You soon reach a junction with the Waterline Trail (also called the Red Trail). Continue straight ahead. If you're here in late spring or early summer, keep an eye out for yellow wood violets (see p. 212).

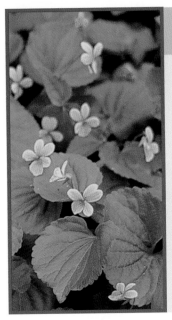

Yellow Wood Violet
(Viola glabella)

Yellow wood violets, also known as stream violets, have heart-shaped leaves and flowers with five petals. The lower petal usually has purple lines pointing down.

Violets are especially interesting because of how they spread their seeds. Whereas seeds from most plants are spread either by the wind, by water or by animals, violets spread their seeds by literally exploding.

What happens is that the capsule that the seeds sit inside gets drier and drier until finally the capsule splits. The seeds get thrown into the air and eventually land on the forest floor. There, they can germinate, set down roots and grow into another yellow wood violet.

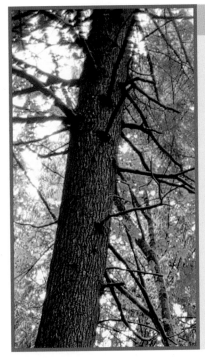

Snags

These old trees may be dead, but they are still important to the life of the forest in many ways. When a tree like this one dies, it creates a space in the forest canopy. Light can then get through and perhaps shine on trees, such as Douglas-fir, that don't grow well in shade. The light will also help smaller trees, shrubs and ferns on the forest floor to grow a bit bigger and thus provide more food and shelter for forest creatures.

The dead, decaying wood of the snag also provides food for insects, such as beetles and ants, which in turn are food for woodpeckers. The holes that the woodpeckers make when they're looking for insects get used by other birds and mammals.

About 15 minutes along, the terrain on either side of the trees gets marshier. Not much farther is your first glimpse of Lost Lake, but go just a bit farther to the junction with the Interlaken Trail. Now go left to a good viewpoint of Lost Lake. There are benches here where you can rest and have a snack.

When you're ready to move on, continue straight ahead past the open meadow and Lost Creek. At the East Gate sign, keep going straight. A few minutes later is a junction with a bench. Go right and, just a few steps farther, look on the left side of the trail for a big old snag (see p. 212).

In a couple of minutes you will come to another junction. Continue straight ahead. At the next junction, about 10 minutes later, is a signboard and map. Take the Waterline Trail on the farthest right. The path meanders alongside lots of vine maple, snags and the occasional fire hydrant. Another 10 minutes later is a junction with the Owl Trail (also part of the Red Trail). Go left.

At the end of Owl Trail, go left. You're now on the trail you started on. A few steps will bring you to Mundy Creek, the sports field and the parking lot.

Lost Lake

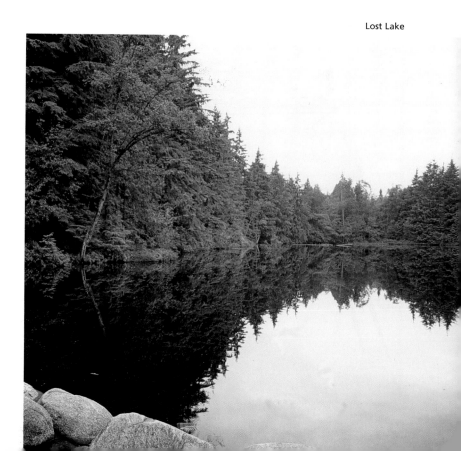

Colony Farm

Length: 5 km

Time needed: 2 to 2.5 hours

Season: Year-round

Rating: Easy

Dogs: Yes, on leash

Stroller-friendly: Yes

Washrooms: Outhouses at parking lot

Highlights: Swallows, Coquitlam River, chicory, coyotes

Access: Take Lougheed Highway to Coquitlam. Between the Cape Horn Interchange and Riverview Hospital, look for Colony Farm Road on the south. Turn right onto it and follow the road to its end. Park in the gravel parking lot on the left.

Driving time: 40 minutes

In the midst of Coquitlam lies Colony Farm, one of the newest regional parks in the Greater Vancouver Regional District. It is a virtual island of green amid growing suburban development. At one time, the land here was farmed. Now, it has reverted to grassland, forest, marsh and riverside habitat that provides food and shelter for a variety of animals.

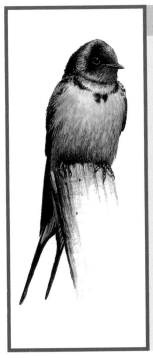

Swallows

Six species of swallow can be seen at Colony Farm. Two species—the bank swallow and cliff swallow—are not very common. The other species—tree swallows, violet-green swallows, northern rough-winged swallows and barn swallows (illustrated)—can almost always be spotted in spring and summer.

Swallows eat all kinds of flying insects, including beetles, ants, wasps, flies, moths and, perhaps best of all, mosquitoes. They have specialized feathers around their mouths, called facial bristles, which are believed to increase sensitivity to the area, like whiskers on a cat.

Swallows spend a lot of time flying. Not only do they eat on the fly, they also take baths on the fly. When flying close to a pond or lake, swallows will dip into the water and use their tail to spray water over their backs. Then they shake the feathers to get out all the dust, oil and nits that might be tucked beneath.

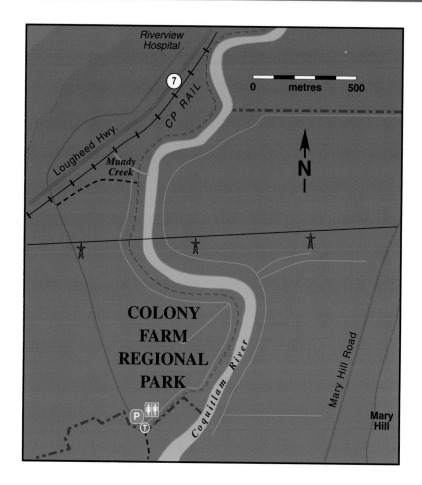

From the parking area, walk southeast to the dyke trail. Part of the
Coquitlam Indian Reserve lies on the right-hand side. On the left is a
ditch that's popular with ducks of all kinds.

If you're here in late summer or early autumn, you'll also notice blackberries everywhere. The blackberries are a perfect example of the mixture
of native and introduced plant life found at Colony Farm. One type of
blackberry, called trailing blackberry, is native to southwestern BC; another, called Himalayan blackberry, was introduced from India via England.
Both species grow here and have delicious berries—and sharp prickles. The
Himalayan blackberry has larger leaves, thicker stems and bigger thorns.

Birds love blackberry thickets, no matter what kind. Some birds eat the
berries. Others find shelter within the tangles of blackberry vines. It's just
one of the features of Colony Farm that attracts more than 150 species
of birds.

One of the best shows going in spring and summer are the aerobatic manoeuvres performed by the swallows (see p. 214) as they swoop and soar above the fields catching insects on the fly.

As the dyke trail continues, curving to a view of the big Mary Hill development, see if you can spot a familiar garden plant alongside the trail. Sweet peas, with their purple, pink and white blossoms, grow here, a hint of the park's farming past.

On the far right, the Coquitlam River scoots by. Not much farther, a newly built bridge spans the water.

Stay on the western dyke and continue deeper into the park, where you'll likely see and hear more and more birds. In autumn or winter, you might see red-tailed hawks hunting for small rodents or great blue herons stalking the ditches for small fish and frogs. Spring and summer are the best times to see a wide variety of birds, including brightly coloured American goldfinches, lazuli buntings and western tanagers.

The Coquitlam River

The Coquitlam River starts amid the snow and ice of the mountains that make up the Pitt-Coquitlam Divide. The meltwater comes tumbling downhill and fills Coquitlam Lake—one of the sources of drinking water for the Lower Mainland.

The river then continues its journey south past gravel-mining operations, where it picks up silt and debris, and past lots of urban development that has paved over many feeder creeks and creeksides. The river usually flows pretty muddy by the time it gets to Colony Farm.

Because of those problems, the Coquitlam River was named the third most endangered river in BC in 2001 by the Outdoor Recreation Council. It's not just the river itself that's in trouble, but also the fish that live there. Salmon and trout can't live in waters that have too much silt in them and so runs of chinook, pink and sockeye salmon that used to be in the Coquitlam have all been wiped out.

Community volunteers have been working hard to restore the fish stocks to the river, but more needs to be done—by federal, provincial and local governments as well as the community.

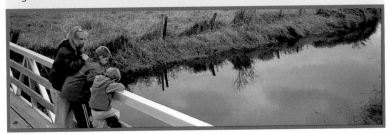

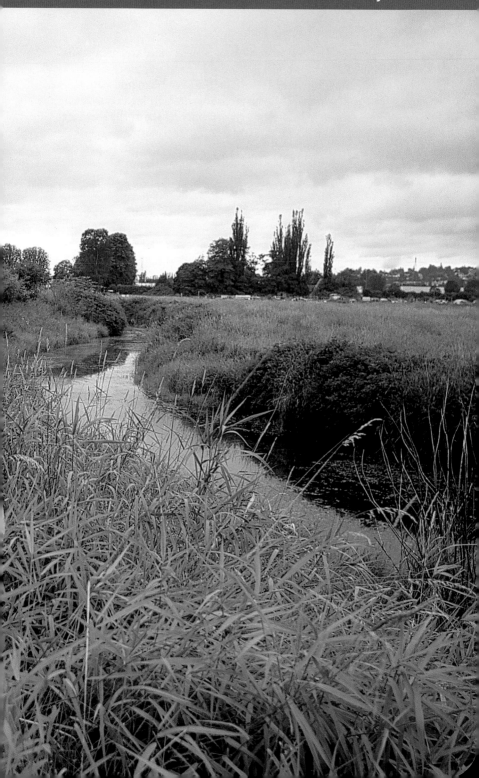

At the next bend of the trail, look for a plant called chicory that has beautiful blue flowers. (It's only here in spring and summer.)

Not much farther up the trail is a slough and an old pump station. The old pilings are now festooned with rows of grass, purple loosestrife and other plants. And an old wooden weir is farther up the ditch. These are all remnants of the park's farming past.

Chicory *(Cichorium intybus)*

Chicory isn't native to BC. Originally, it came from Europe. Now it's established itself all over the world.

The leaves have been used in salads since the days of ancient Egypt. The leaves also can be processed to make a blue dye. The roots, which have a kind of caramel taste, can be steamed and eaten as a vegetable, or they can be roasted and used as a coffee substitute.

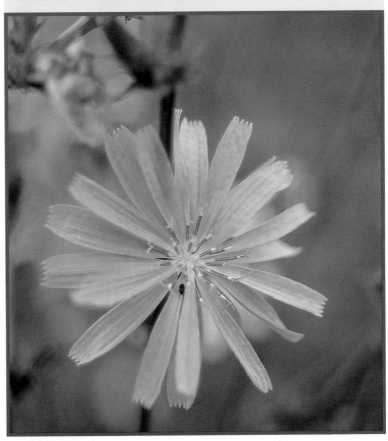

These days, the ditches are used by animals such as beavers, muskrats and river otters. Deer and black bears are also sometimes seen here, but the most familiar mammal around is the coyote.

The dyke trail passes under some powerlines. On the left is Mundy Creek. On the right is a lone Sitka spruce tree. Soon the path parallels Lougheed Highway. At this point, you can turn around and go back to the trailhead. The trail does continue a bit farther to the Pitt River Road, but you just get closer to the roar of traffic.

Coyote (Canis latrans)

The coyote belongs to the same genus of animals as dogs do—*Canis*. A couple hundred years ago, the coyote was only found on the prairies and deserts of North America. Now, it is found just about everywhere in Canada and the US, including cities.

Although the coyote prefers to eat meat, it will eat just about anything that's around. In urban areas like ours, most of the coyote's diet is made up of small animals such as rabbits and rodents (rats, mice, etc.) But it will also scavenge on animals killed by other animals or by people (roadkill, for example.) As well, a coyote will eat berries, other fruit, insects and birds.

Coyotes will usually avoid people and with good reason. For many, many years, coyotes have been killed using poison, traps and guns. People usually kill coyotes because they prey on animals such as chickens and sheep.

But even though there are some problems, coyotes help us, too. They eat rodents that eat grain and sometimes carry disease. And coyotes help get rid of dead animals whose bodies might otherwise rot and cause problems of their own.

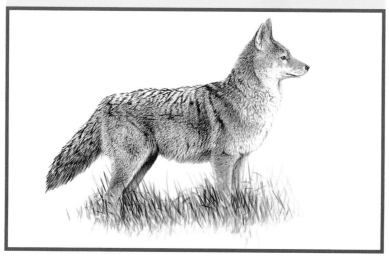

Minnekhada

Length: 3-km loop

Time needed: 1.5 to 2 hours

Season: Year-round

Rating: Easy; one short uphill section

Dogs: Yes, on leash

Stroller-friendly: No

Washrooms: At parking lot trailhead; at picnic area

Highlights: Red alder, beavers, moss, turtles

Access: Take Lougheed Highway to Port Coquitlam. Turn north on Coast Meridian Road and follow the green and yellow park signs to the Quarry Road entrance (Right on Apel Drive, right on Victoria Drive until it forks left and becomes the gravel of Quarry Road.) The park entrance is on the right, roughly 3.5 kilometres from the fork.

Driving time: 45 minutes

Once a country estate, Minnekhada's marsh, forest and rocky knolls are now a park, filled with a variety of plants and animals. Our route scoots along dykes and trails for a close-up look at some of the park's inhabitants and features a short scramble to a knoll that offers a bigger picture of the area.

From the Quarry Road parking lot, walk along the trail lined with salmonberries to a junction. Then go left and follow that trail a bit farther to another junction. Go right to follow the Meadow Trail.

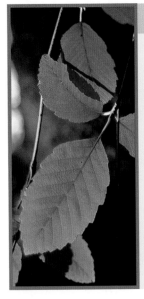

Red Alder *(Alnus rubra)*

Alder trees are common all over southwestern BC. They're one of the first trees to grow when land has been cleared by logging or fire. They grow very quickly, but they don't live for very long. Alder trees are considered to be old when they reach 50 or 60 years of age. Compare that to trees that can live more than 1000 years.

Alder trees are very important to the health of the forest. They turn nutrient-poor dirt into rich dirt. In the roots of an alder tree live bacteria that remove nitrogen from the air and 'fix' it in a form that is useful to plants.

Each season, the alder drops its leaves, providing more nutrients for the soil. By the time the alder dies, the ground has been nicely conditioned for other kinds of trees to grow.

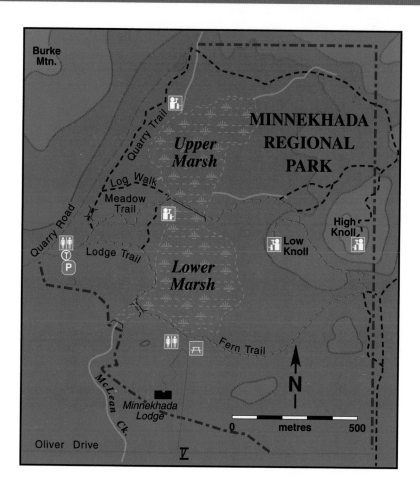

As you walk along, notice the different species of trees. Some are vine maple with their skinny, twisty trunks and tiny maple leaves. Others are red alder (see p. 220 and photo on p. 222).

Continue along the trail as it heads uphill and into a grove of conifers, or cone-bearing trees, such as cedar, fir and hemlock. You soon come to a junction. Go left and down a rocky, rooty trail to the next signpost. Then go right to the marsh and a little bridge.

If you look to the Upper Marsh, you should be able to see some beaver lodges—what look like big piles of sticks lying in the water (see p. 223).

Walk along the dyke that separates the Upper and Lower marshes. At the end of the dyke, the trail climbs through cool, open forest. After a while, the trail descends through rocks and roots, then climbs gently alongside a stream and a beautiful lush grove of ferns, shrubs and trees.

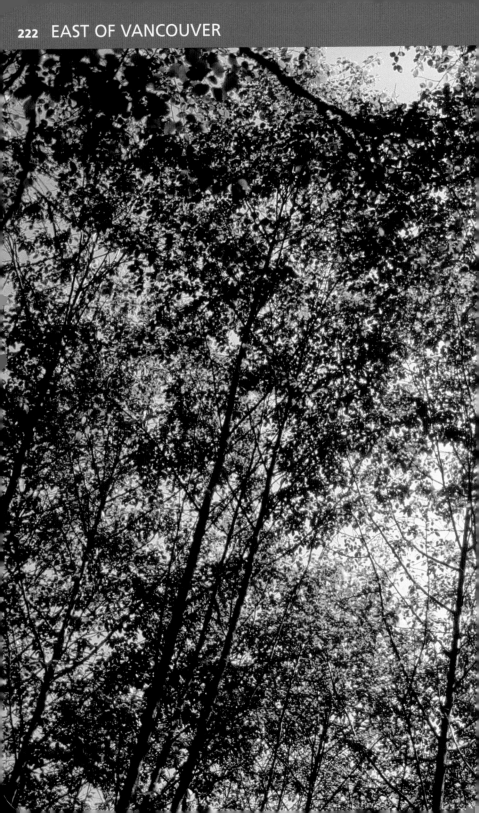

Beaver Lodges

A beaver's lodge protects it from predators—coyotes, wolves, black bears, bobcats and even eagles will eat beavers. Inside the lodge the beaver's nesting chamber is above the level of the water, so the beaver stays dry. The roof is made of twigs, branches and small trees that have been chewed down by beavers. Before winter, a layer of mud is added to make the roof even stronger.

Beavers are very strong animals. They have a sturdy skeleton and strong muscles to haul all the trees they bring down and to build dams and lodges. Their teeth are also big and strong—they can chew through trees more than a metre in diameter. Beavers' teeth continue to grow as long as they live.

A beaver's big, flat tail acts as a rudder to help a beaver steer when it swims, and it acts as an alarm when a beaver slaps its tail on the water.

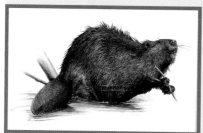

Sometimes the beavers here try to make a dam just under the bridge you're standing on. But the ducks that live in the Lower Marsh also need water, so people from Ducks Unlimited usually come and clear out all the branches, mud and muck.

Beaver lodge and dam

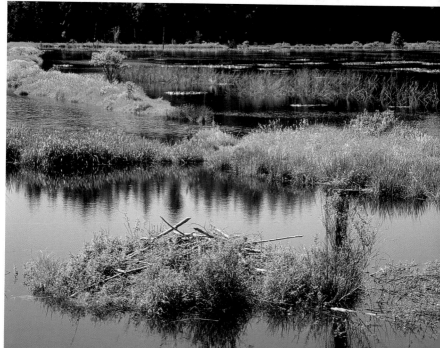

A few minutes later is a trail junction. Go right toward Low Knoll. A few minutes later is another signpost. Go right again. And a couple of minutes later you'll reach a third signpost. Go right. Another couple of minutes brings you to Low Knoll—a good spot for lunch or a snack.

From Low Knoll there are views of the Lower Marsh, Burke Mountain and, in the distance, the North Arm of the Fraser River. When you're ready to move on, retrace your steps to the last signpost and go right. The trail descends through a section that is lush with green—ferns, vine maple, Oregon grape (see p. 187), cedar, salal and moss.

Moss

There are about 700 species of moss in coastal BC. They come in a range of colours, from yellow to red to black, but most mosses are green.

Although moss might not look too exciting—it doesn't have flowers or a nice smell—it is interesting in a couple of ways. Take, for example, the way that moss reproduces. Unlike some other plants that reproduce using seeds, moss uses spores.

On most mosses, the spores are stored in a tiny capsule at the end of a skinny little stalk that makes it look like the moss has a whole bunch of little antennae. When the spores mature, the capsule pops open and the spores are carried away. If a spore falls on someplace damp—the ground, a stump, a fallen tree, even a rock—it grows into moss.

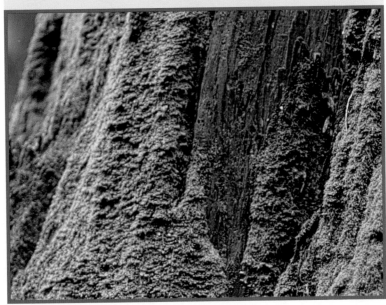

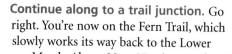

Continue along to a trail junction. Go right. You're now on the Fern Trail, which slowly works its way back to the Lower Marsh. About 20 to 25 minutes of walking brings you to a picnic area with washrooms. Stay right to go along the south end of the Lower Marsh. Now it's time to take a look at the Lower Marsh and its inhabitants. Here you can see all species of birds—ducks, swallows, herons, hawks—as well as muskrats, frogs and turtles.

Stay on the trail as it leads back into the woods. About 250 metres in is a trail junction. Stay to the left to follow the Lodge Trail back to the parking area.

Red-tailed hawk

Turtles

One of the best places to look for turtles is where there are rocks or pieces of wood sticking out above the surface of the water. Turtles love to crawl up there so they can lie in the sun. Sometimes you can see turtles stacked on top of one another when there aren't enough rocks or wood for them to lie on.

Although there are three native species of turtles in BC, the turtles in Minnekhada Regional Park are not among them. These turtles are a species called red-eared sliders (*Trachemys scripta* ssp. *elegans*). They're the same kind of tiny little turtles you sometimes see in pet stores. When these turtles grow bigger, a lot of people decide they don't want them as pets anymore, so they let them go in the nearest pond.

That might sound like a nice thing to do for the turtle, but it's not a good thing for some of the other creatures that live in the pond: turtles eat the same plants that the native animals need.

Pitt Wildlife Marsh

Length: 6-km loop

Time needed: 2.5 to 3 hours

Season: Year-round

Rating: Moderate; flat but long

Dogs: Yes, on leash

Stroller-friendly: No

Washrooms: Outhouses near trailhead

Highlights: Pitt Lake, grasses, damselflies

Access: Take Lougheed Highway to Pitt Meadows. At the first stoplight after the Pitt River Bridge, turn left onto Dewdney Trunk Road. At Harris Road, turn left to follow the sign for Pitt Lake. At McNeil, turn right. At Rannie Road, turn left and follow it to the end at Grant Narrows.

Driving time: 1 hour

Pitt Wildlife Marsh can be a great escape from the hustle and bustle of the city. Most of the dyke-top trails are flat and open allowing for big views of Pitt Lake and the surrounding mountains. But the trails also provide good viewing for things closer at hand—birds, insects, wildflowers and greenery of all kinds.

From the parking area, head east to the locked gate and the gravel dyke-top path. If you look directly across the Narrows, you can see Katzie Reserve No. 4. The people of the Katzie First Nation have lived in this area for hundreds of years. They fished for sturgeon and salmon, hunted deer, seal and ducks and gathered all kinds of plants and berries in the surrounding marshes.

Pitt Marsh

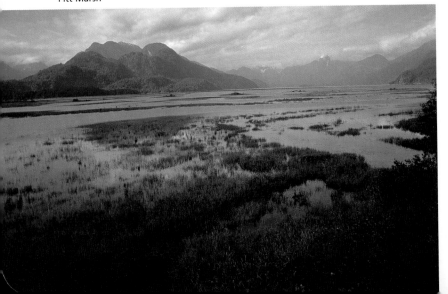

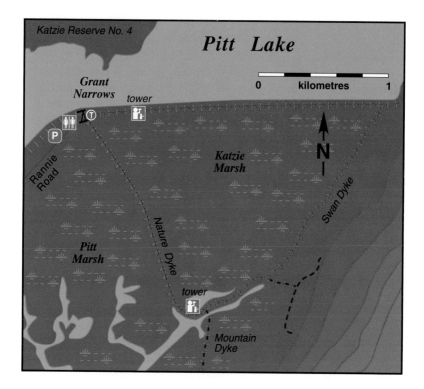

About 10 minutes of walking brings you to an observation tower. Climb up and take a look at the surrounding views.

As you continue east along the path, be sure to check out the pilings in the near distance. Ospreys build nests on some of the pilings—one of the few places in the Lower Mainland where ospreys breed. For a place to be

Pitt Lake

A long time ago, Pitt Lake used to be a fjord. A fjord is actually a Norwegian term that describes a long, steep-walled arm of the sea that reaches inland. Originally, glaciers scraped out these troughs. There are fjords up and down the coast of BC. The closest fjord to Vancouver is Indian Arm.

A long time ago, Pitt Lake was part of the sea. But year after year, the Fraser River deposited silt, sand and gravel at the south end of the fjord until finally it was pretty much closed off. Then it became a lake.

Pitt Lake is now what is called a tidal lake. The height of the water is still affected by the ocean tides going out and coming in. That's because the Pacific Ocean is so near that it raises and lowers the height of the Fraser River and the Pitt River as the tide comes in and goes out. That, in turn, affects the lake.

just right it needs tall trees—or pilings—on which to build nests and an abundance of fish for ospreys to hunt and eat.

On the right of the trail is Pitt Marsh—a haven for birds of all kinds. What kinds of birds you'll see depends to some extent on the season. In winter, the marsh is home to trumpeter swans, ring-necked ducks and lots of other waterfowl. In spring and summer, flycatchers, vireos and warblers flit about. And in autumn, birds on their southward migration stop to feed and rest.

The brush on either side of the trail is cut during spring and summer months. But you can still see the occasional wildflower, including hardhack, pussytoes and fireweed.

About 45 minutes from the start is the end of the lakeside dyke. Go right onto Swan Dyke, named for the trumpeter swans that are common here in winter and spring. It could just as easily be called Goose Dyke, as you'll notice all sorts of goose poop and goose feathers lying around. Occasionally, you might even see the remnants of a goose and coyote tussle—a fight the coyote almost always wins.

If you're here in summer, be sure to scan the grass and the shoreline for another kind of winged creature that lives here in great numbers— damselflies (see p. 229).

About 20 to 25 minutes of walking brings you to the end of Swan Dyke. Go right. On a hot day in summer, you'll be happy to reach this point with its shade from the nearby cottonwood and alder trees. Look to the marsh on the other side of the trees and you'll see beaver lodges. In spring and summer, it's easy to see the fresh branches that have been added to the top of the lodge.

About 10 minutes of walking will bring you to another observation tower. Go up for a 360-degree view of the marsh and great views of the distant peaks. If you're here in spring or early summer, you may also see swallow nests built under the eaves of the tower's roof.

Grasses

Grasses don't usually get noticed as much as other plants. They don't have pretty flowers, nice scents or edible berries. They just kind of hang out in the background. But grasses are important to all kinds of wildlife. Some animals depend on grasses for food. Others depend on grasses to build nests and provide shelter.

Among the kinds of grasses you'll see here in summer are bluejoint (*Calamagrostis canadensis*), reed canary grass (*Phalaris arundinacea*) and wood reedgrass (*Cinna latifolia*). All were used by coastal First Nations peoples in basket-making.

Once down, continue past the tower along the Nature Dyke. In summer, the trail is heavily overgrown with all kinds of vegetation. It's still walkable, but you'll be going in single file. Among the greenery here are lots of grasses (see p. 228).

Eventually, the path widens and brings you back to the boat launch area. All you need to do is head left to reach the parking lot.

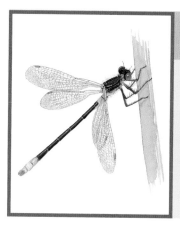

Damselflies (Order Zygoptera)

There are a couple of good ways to tell damselflies (such as the common spreadwing, illustrated) apart from dragonflies. First, damselflies are generally smaller than dragonflies. Second is how they hold their wings. If the wings are straight out to the side, they're dragonflies. But if they hold their wings together above their body, they're damselflies.

Grasses

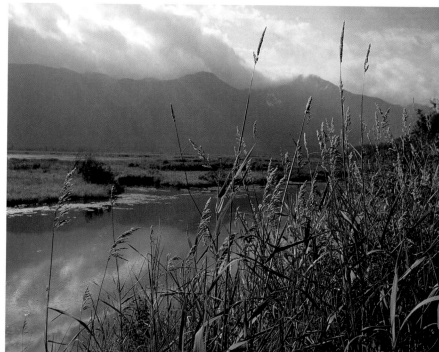

Widgeon Falls

Length: 6 km

Time needed: 2.5 to 3 hours (plus 3 to 4 hours paddling)

Season: Year-round

Rating: Moderate; elevation gain of 100 m

Dogs: Yes, on leash

Stroller-friendly: No

Washrooms: Outhouses at Grant Narrows, Widgeon Campsite and upper falls

Highlights: Muskrats, Widgeon Creek, deer fern, potholes, waterfalls

Access: Take Lougheed Highway to Pitt Meadows. At the first stoplight after the Pitt River Bridge, turn left onto Dewdney Trunk Road. At Harris Road, turn left to follow the sign for Pitt Lake. At McNeil, turn right. At Rannie Road, turn left and follow it to the end at Grant Narrows.

Note: You need a canoe or kayak to access trailhead. From June to September, canoes can be rented at Grant Narrows from Ayla Canoe Rentals; call or check the website for hours and rates (p. 248). It's best to wear waterproof sandals or old running shoes for canoeing and bring hiking boots along.

Driving time: 1 hour

The hike to Widgeon Falls begins with a lazy paddle up Widgeon Slough through marshlands dotted with ducks, herons, hawks and many other species of bird. It continues along a path that rambles from sweet-smelling forest to creekside, finally ending at beautiful Widgeon Falls.

Paddle across the narrows, being sure to watch for power boats and jet skis that also use the area. As you paddle into Widgeon Slough, look for some of the birds that live here, such as great blue herons, catbirds and swallows. You'll also need to watch for the signs to point you toward the campsite and the start of the hiking trail. (Ask for a map and directions when you rent the canoe.)

Widgeon Slough

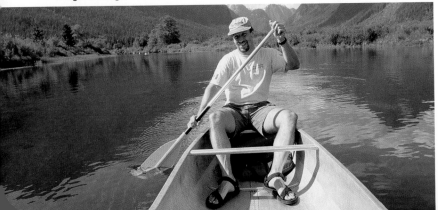

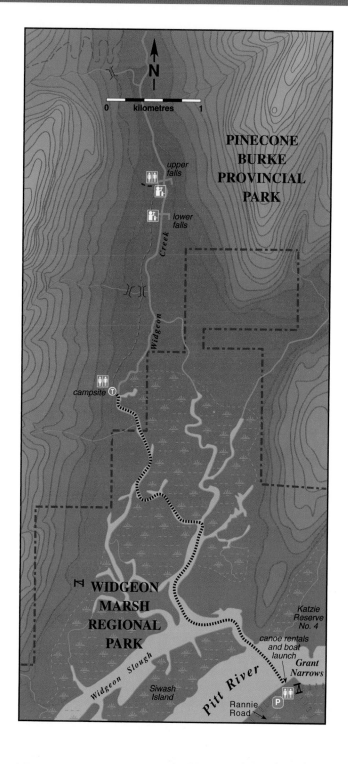

N

0 kilometres 1

PINECONE
BURKE
PROVINCIAL
PARK

upper
falls

lower
falls

Widgeon

Creek

campsite T

WIDGEON
MARSH
REGIONAL
PARK

Katzie
Reserve
No. 4

canoe rentals
and boat
launch

Grant
Narrows

Widgeon Slough

Siwash
Island

Pitt River

Rannie
Road

A while later, when you're paddling along some of the smaller channels of the slough, look at the muddy banks for big holes—burrows where muskrats live.

Muskrat (Ondatra zibethicus)

Muskrats are brown, about the size of a cat, and have a long rat-like tail that helps them swim through the water. Muskrats usually eat plants growing in or near the water, but if they find fish, frogs, turtles, fresh-water clams or mussels, they'll eat those, too.

Muskrats can swim for at least 100 metres underwater and even stay under for as long as 17 minutes.

Muskrats, like beavers, can also build houses. But here in Widgeon Slough, they tend to make burrows in the riverbanks. Most of the time, the entrance to the burrows is underwater, but because the water level is affected by the tide, you can sometimes see the holes where muskrats go in and come out.

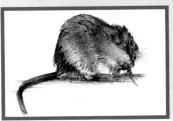

If the water gets too low, or if a muskrat can't find a riverbank that's big enough to dig a burrow into, it will build a house of grasses, cattails and bulrushes, mud and muck. But although beaver lodges can last a long time, most muskrat houses only last for one winter.

Once you're reached the campsite, carry the canoe high enough out of the water so it won't drift away if the tide comes in. Then, change into your hiking shoes and walk toward an old gravel road. About 250 metres up the road on the right is a sign that marks the trail to the falls.

Follow the orange diamond-shaped markers along the trail as it passes through a forest of mostly second-growth hemlock trees and old stumps. In spring and summer, there are lots of ferns, foamflowers and salmonberries. Occasionally, you can look up to see a big beautiful moss-covered maple tree.

About 10 to 15 minutes of walking brings you to a section of boardwalk and a grove of Sitka spruce trees. At the end of the boardwalk, look for a wooden beaver, named Chizzel, who was carved by a local sculptor.

As the trail continues through the forest, you might see or hear some of the birds that live here—blue Steller's jays, red-topped woodpeckers and sapsuckers. Be sure to watch your step as the trail can be muddy at times.

A bigleaf maple and a Sitka spruce tree straddle the trail where the 1 kilometre marker is. Another five minutes of hiking brings you to a new bridge. This creek is just one of many small side creeks and streams that flow into

Widgeon Creek—just on your right. Depending on what time of year you're here, Widgeon Creek may be a thin green ribbon of water running through a bed of rocks or a wide churning creek that fills the whole channel.

The water that comes down Widgeon Creek starts about 7 kilometres upstream at Widgeon Lake. The water in the lake comes mostly from melting snow. In springtime, when much snow is melting, a lot more water comes down the creek. In summer, when most of the snow up high has melted, there's less water to come down the creek.

The trail goes up a little rise and along a 10-metre high creek bank. From here, you can see some of the places where Widgeon Creek forms beautiful green pools. Not much farther, there's a little clearing at creek-side with some logs and shade where you can take a short break.

The trail goes up a short steepish hill, then levels, then descends a wooden stairway to a hillside covered in deer ferns.

A bit farther along the trail is another uphill section, this one on a wooden staircase. About 15 to 20 minutes later, you'll come to the Lower Falls. In some places, there are small swimming holes where the water isn't too powerful. So, you can sit with your socks and shoes off and soak your toes, or if you're brave enough maybe you could even go for a swim. Just be careful when you're walking around. The rocks can be slippery,

Deer Fern *(Blechnum spicant)*

Lots of different species of ferns grow in the forests of southwestern BC, including one called a deer fern. But how do you tell a deer fern from other kinds of ferns?

Deer fern fronds are shaped like feathers—they're narrow at the bottom, then get a bit fatter in the middle and then get narrow again at the top. They're skinnier than other ferns, such as sword ferns and bracken ferns. And they have two kinds of fronds—one kind grows in clumps close to the ground, the second kind grows straight up and is usually even skinnier.

These ferns are important food for deer in some places, especially during winter when not as many plants grow on the forest floor.

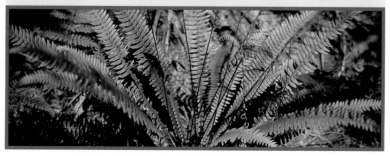

whether they're wet or mossy. Parents will have to decide whether or not their children can go in.

The upper falls (see p. 235) are about a 5 to 10 minute walk farther up the trail. Here, you can see even better how the water has pounded the rocks over years and years and years.

Once you've taken a good look around, had a snack and some water and rested your feet, all you need to do is return to the trail and retrace your steps to the canoe.

Potholes

Try to imagine all the different ways that the constant force of the river has eroded the rocks here. In some places, it has made rock that used to be rough and jagged into rock that is smooth and round. And in other places it has made potholes.

What happens to make a pothole? Well, the rock of the streambed is not smooth and has many irregularities in it. In some places, the rock forms a higher shelf; in others, it forms a shallow dip. Loose rocks—from pebbles to boulders—can get trapped in those dips by the fast-flowing currents above. But they don't sit still. The current, instead of moving the rocks farther downstream, moves the rocks around and around the dip. And as they go around and around over the years, the depression gets deeper and deeper until it becomes a pothole.

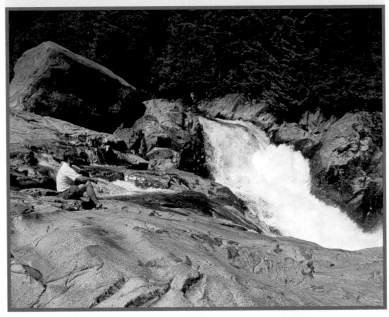

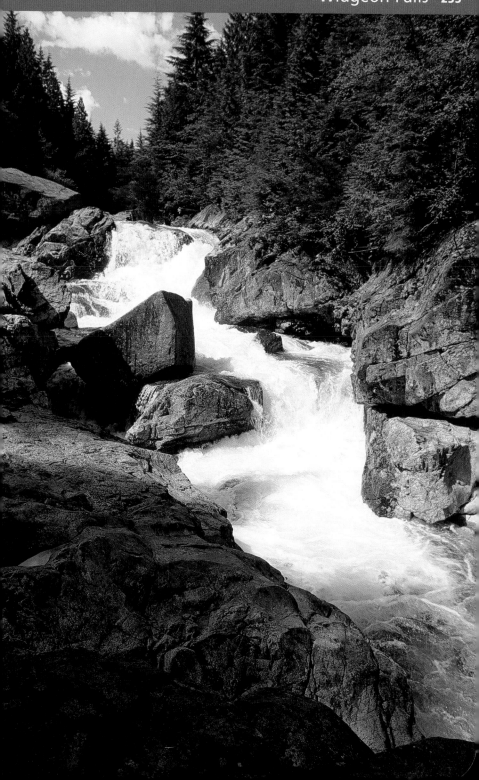

Kanaka Creek

Length: 3.5-km loop

Time needed: 1.5 to 2 hours

Season: Year-round

Rating: Moderate; short but hilly

Dogs: Yes, on leash

Stroller-friendly: All-terrain stroller only

Washrooms: At picnic area

Highlights: Rosy twistedstalk, waterfalls, tailed frogs

Access: Take Lougheed Highway east to Maple Ridge. At the first traffic light in Maple Ridge, turn left to take the Dewdney Trunk Road. Follow it east to 252nd Street, then turn right. Follow the road to its end and park in the lot next to a playing field.

Driving time: 1 hour

Kanaka Creek is one of the best-kept secrets of the Greater Vancouver Regional Parks system. And even though it's a bit farther to go than most of the urban parks, it's worth the drive. In total, the park protects 12 kilometres of Kanaka Creek, but there aren't yet trails through all of it. This hike covers some of the trails in the Cliff Falls portion of the park.

From the parking area, walk south past the playing field to a sign that shows the area's trails. Go downhill and straight until you reach a bridge. Before crossing the North Fork bridge, go right to a viewpoint of Cliff Falls.

Once you've had a look at this pretty cascade, return to the bridge and cross. You can see Kanaka Creek rushing below as well as the top of the falls. At the end of the bridge, go right and down the set of stairs to another viewpoint of more waterfalls. Take a look, but heed the signs and stay behind the fence. Also notice the rock here—it's different from the granite you might be used to seeing. It's sandstone.

Continue walking along the trail as it heads uphill. At the top of the hill, go right and over the bridge. Although you can't see them from here,

Sandstone, Kanaka Creek

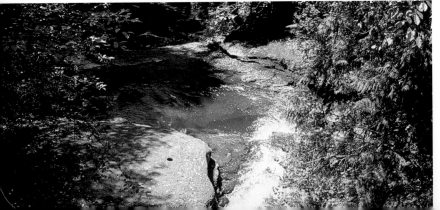

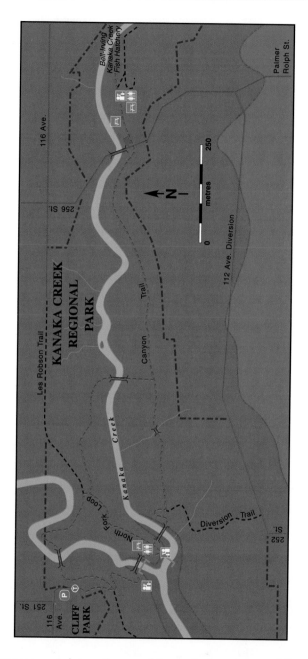

there are some very interesting—and increasingly rare—amphibians that live in the water below. They're called tailed frogs (see p. 239).

The trail climbs uphill past salmonberry bushes and, in summer, tiny wildflowers. At the top of the hill, go left past the yellow posts. Cross a little bridge and amble along the canyon top. You soon cross another small bridge over a tributary stream of Kanaka Creek.

After a downhill section, you'll come upon a huge nurse log. Ferns, huckleberry, moss, vine maple and western hemlock can all be found growing here. Be sure to look for one other plant growing here, called rosy twistedstalk (see p. 239).

The trail climbs up and away from the creek and through the lush understorey and second-growth forest. Cross one more small bridge and you'll soon come to a trail junction. Go straight for another 0.75 kilometres and cross 256th Avenue to reach the Bell-Irving Hatchery.

Juvenile salmon and trout are raised here. You can see them most times of the year, and there are free tours most days between 2 and 3 p.m. Call (604) 462-8643 to be sure the hatchery is open the day you want to go.

When you're done at the hatchery, retrace your steps to the trail junction. Go right and down some steps to a viewpoint of the creek. Then, continue down farther to the creekside. There's a small sandbar next to the bridge where you can take off your shoes and soak your toes.

Cross the metal bridge and go left. The trail climbs uphill at first, then levels. This spot is one of the places in the park to see a Steller's jay.

You soon come to a junction. You could go right up the road to follow the North Fork Loop Trail back to the starting point. Or you could take the slightly shorter route, and go left to return to the picnic area by the waterfalls.

Nurse log

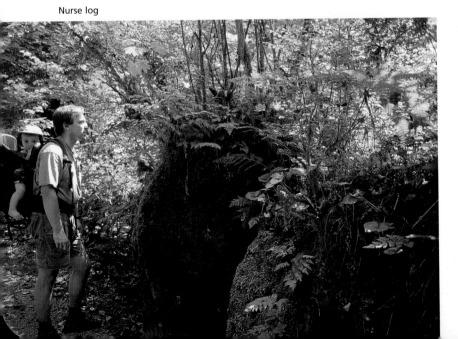

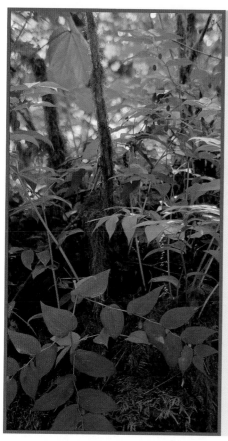

Rosy Twistedstalk
(Streptopus roseus)

Depending on the time of year, you might see a plant that has tiny, pink, bell-shaped flowers or small, red berries.

Rosy twistedstalk is one of three kinds of twistedstalk found in coastal BC. But if you look at the stalk, or stem, you'll notice it isn't actually twisted. So where did the name come from? There is a similar plant called clasping twistedstalk that has a stem that zigs and zags and looks kind of twisted.

The berries of all three kinds of twistedstalk are not edible. In fact, most BC First Nations peoples considered them poisonous and gave them names such as 'witch-berries,' 'grizzly berries' or 'frog-berries.'

Tailed Frog *(Ascaphus truei)*

Most frogs like their water warm and still. That's not the case with tailed frogs, which prefer cold, clear, fast-flowing forest streams. They lay eggs in the stream, attaching them to the underside of rocks. Tailed frog tadpoles have a special mouth that acts like a suction cup so they can attach themselves to rocks in the current. As adults, tailed frogs leave the water to search the forest floor for food—insects and bugs of all different kinds.

Tailed frogs aren't very big as frogs go. Adults range from the size of a quarter to the size of a small lime.

Tailed frogs are considered a blue-listed species in BC. That means that they're not yet an endangered species, but scientists are concerned that these frogs are vulnerable to extinction because of loss of habitat or water pollution.

Gold Creek Falls

Distance: 5.5 km return

Time needed: 2.5 to 3 hours

Season: Year-round

Rating: Moderate

Dogs: Yes, on leash

Stroller-friendly: All-terrain stroller only

Washrooms: Outhouses at trailhead

Highlights: Erratic boulders, giant stumps, mountain views, waterfalls

Access: Take Lougheed Highway east to Maple Ridge. At the first traffic light in Maple Ridge, turn left to take the Dewdney Trunk Road. Follow it east to 232nd Street, then turn left. Look for the blue and white Golden Ears Provincial Park signs and follow them to the park entrance. Keep going another 14 kilometres to the Gold Creek day-use area.

Driving time: 1 hour

From the parking area, head down one of the connecting paths toward the creek. The wide main trail heads east into classic rainforest. Even in winter, it looks green here because of all the moss and lichen.

Continue along the trail, shifting your attention to all the different species of tree. Even if you don't know the names of the different kinds, just try to notice the differences in bark or needles or leaves. Most of the coniferous trees, which have needles and cones, are Douglas-fir, western hemlock and western redcedar. The biggest of these trees are about 70 years old. But you can still see stumps from even bigger trees that grew here before.

Soon, you should hear the rushing waters of Gold Creek. Just a few minutes later, you'll be walking next to it. Around this same point, you'll get the first peeks at some of the mountains surrounding the valley. The trail levels and leaves the rainforest to enter a wide-open area with red alder trees and some bigleaf maples. From here, you have great views of four peaks across the creek.

Gold Creek view

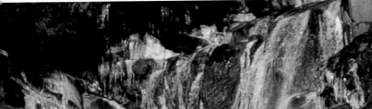

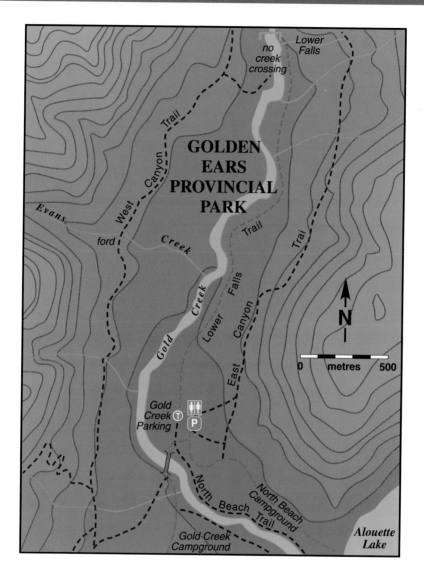

Now it's time to continue along the trail and into the rainforest again. You'll cross a number of creeks over small—and sometimes slippery—wooden bridges. Before you know it, you'll hear the roar of the waterfalls ahead. Next, you'll see spray and then you'll see the Lower Falls.

Follow the trail a bit farther and higher to where there is a good viewpoint. Remember not to go beyond the fence—it's slippery and steep.

Once you've absorbed enough spray, enough falls and enough tranquillity, simply head back down the trail with all its views of mountain and forest before returning home.

UBC Malcolm Knapp Research Forest

Length: 2.5-km loop

Time needed: 1.5 to 2 hours

Season: Year-round

Rating: Easy to moderate

Dogs: Not allowed

Stroller-friendly: All-terrain stroller only

Washrooms: Outhouses near parking area

Highlights: Steam donkey, North Alouette River, red huckleberry, arboretum

Access: Take Lougheed Highway east to Maple Ridge. Where Dewdney Trunk Road meets the Lougheed, turn left and follow Dewdney Trunk to 232nd Street. Here, turn left and drive 3.5 kilometres to a fork in the road. Take the right fork, Silver Valley Road, for 1.5 kilometres to the parking area at the research forest.

Driving time: 50 minutes

The **UBC Malcolm Knapp Research Forest** is an undiscovered gem in the Fraser Valley that is full of trails and things to see. Even when nearby parks, such as Golden Ears, are overflowing with cars and people, the research forest is usually a cool, quiet place to get away from it all.

From the parking area, go past the gate and up the main road. About 100 metres from the gate, look on the left for an old steam donkey and make a short side trip to check it out.

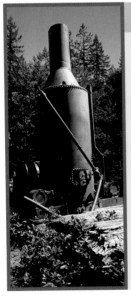

The Steam Donkey

Built by the Empire Company in Vancouver, this steam donkey was one of about 20 used in the 1920s by the Abernethy and Lougheed Logging Company, which logged in the area, including parts of what is now Golden Ears Provincial Park.

The steam donkey was used for something called yarding. A cable would be attached to a downed tree and the steam engine would then reel the cable in, dragging the tree from the forest to a river or a rail line. The trees would then be taken to a mill and cut into lumber and other wood products.

In the 1930s, the logging operations were shut down and the steam donkeys were abandoned. In 1974, this particular donkey was found by some University of BC students on the shores of Pitt Lake. It was restored and moved here.

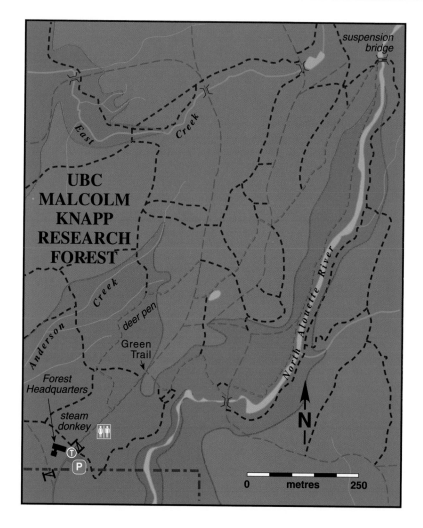

Now, go back to the main road and continue north for another 50 metres. In the distance are some of the snow-covered peaks of Golden Ears Provincial Park—Alouette Mountain, Mount Blanshard and Golden Ears. But also watch on the right for the start of the Green Trail. Then, go right.

About 15 metres farther is a fork; go left toward the sound of the rushing water below. Stay with the trail as it follows along the clifftops above the river. Soon, the trail descends to a gravel road. Go right and to the bridge. Below, the North Alouette River churns through a canyon, complete with a couple of waterfalls.

Now backtrack to the west side of the bridge and look on the right for a trail descending into the forest. You soon come upon a shelter and bench—a nice place to stop and look at the waterfall and have something to drink.

The narrow trail winds through second-growth forest along the river. A short distance farther, it joins a wider path. Go right to continue along the river. Not much farther is a small pebble 'beach.' Have some lunch here or maybe just stick your toes in the water.

When you're ready, continue hiking through lush mixed forest with the occasional stump from trees that were cut down about 80 years ago. Some of the living plants include ferns, salmonberry and huckleberry (see p. 245).

When you pass through a particularly wet, marshy section of the trail, look up to see the stump of what was once a big western redcedar. It gives you an idea of how big the trees here once were.

Soon, the trail emerges to meet another trail. Go right to take a look at a wooden suspension bridge. Then, retrace your steps back to the west side and go up the trail, into the forest and away from the river. The trail is level at first, then goes a bit uphill.

The North Alouette River

The North Alouette River starts as snow high on Alouette Mountain. Along the way, it's joined by other small creeks and streams, growing in size as it passes through the UBC Research Forest. The river heads farther south to about 132nd Avenue and then makes an abrupt turn west to parallel the Alouette River that flows out of Alouette Lake. The two rivers finally join together in Pitt Meadows, just before emptying into the Pitt River. Once there, the waters head a bit farther south to the Fraser River.

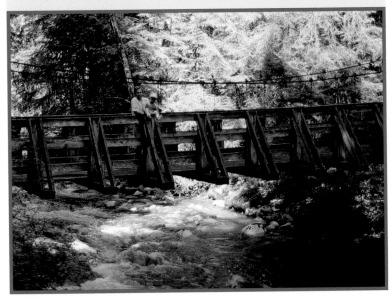

Red Huckleberry *(Vaccinium parvifolium)*

There are actually a couple different species of huckleberry that grow in coastal BC, but red huckleberries are the best known. The little orange-red berries are edible but can be pretty tart.

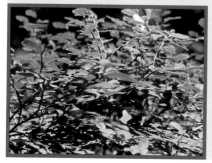

BC's First Nations peoples ate the berries fresh, dried, mashed into cakes or soaked in oil. They also used the berries as fish bait. The branches of the huckleberry bush were used as firewood. The leaves and bark were used to make medicines to help heal sore throats and gums. The leaves were also used to make tea.

You soon come to a junction. Go left. About 100 metres farther is another junction; go straight across the road and continue along the Green Trail. A few minutes later is another junction. Go left again and take a look at some of the signs that tell you about forestry practices such as edge treatment, crown thinning and mechanical thinning.

At the next trail junction is a pretty little pond below. Take a look, then go right. The trail meets a gravel road. You could go left and walk along the gravel road back to the parking area. But for a nicer walk, go right on the gravel road for about 100 metres past a sign explaining white pine blister rust. Look on the left for a trail leading into the woods and follow it.

At the T junction, go left. And, a few minutes later, at the next junction, go left again to reach a bark mulch trail. Here, go right, past a building that was the entrance to a large deer pen. (Researchers have kept deer in the pen in order to find a harmless 'deer repellent' that will keep deer from eating newly planted tree seedlings—a favourite food of deer.) When you come to a T junction, go left and soon, you'll see the old steam donkey (see p. 242).

The parking lot is straight ahead, but take a few minutes to stroll through the arboretum and look at some of the different trees from all over the world. Think of an arboretum as a living tree museum. Plants from many different countries—with their own particular climatic conditions—have been planted here. Signs for most of the trees tell you the common name of the tree, the scientific name of the tree and the country it is native to. The arboretum helps researchers understand how non-native trees can adapt to our climate.

When you've finished, it's just a short walk back to the parking area.

Selected Bibliography

Armstrong, Dr. John. *Vancouver Geology*. Vancouver: Geological Association of Canada, 1990.

Baron, Nancy and Acorn, John. *Birds of Coastal British Columbia*. Edmonton: Lone Pine Publishing, 1997.

Burns, Bill. *Discover Burns Bog*. Vancouver: Hurricane Press, 1997.

Cannings, Richard and Cannings, Sydney. *British Columbia: A Natural History*. Vancouver: Greystone Books, 1996.

Corkran, Charlotte and Thoms, Chris. *Amphibians of Oregon, Washington and British Columbia*. Edmonton: Lone Pine Publishing, 1996.

Ehrlich, Paul, Dobkin, David and Wheye, Darryl. *The Birder's Handbook*. New York: Fireside, 1988.

Klots, Alexander and Klots, Elsie. *1001 Questions Answered About Insects*. New York: Dover, 1977.

McTaggart-Cowan, Ian. *The Mammals of British Columbia*. Victoria: BC Provincial Museum, 1965.

Milne, Lorne and Milne, Margery. *The Audubon Society Field Guide to North American Insects and Spiders*. New York: Alfred A. Knopf, 1980.

Pearson, T. Gilbert, ed. *Birds of America*. Garden City: Garden City Books, 1936.

Pojar, Jim and MacKinnon, Andy, eds. *Plants of Coastal British Columbia*. Vancouver: Lone Pine Publishing, 1994.

Smith, Kathleen, Anderson, Nancy and Beamish, Katherine, eds. *Nature West Coast*. Victoria: Sono Nis Press, 1988.

Sparks, Dawn and Border, Martha. *Echoes Across the Inlet*. North Vancouver: Deep Cove and Area Heritage Association, 1989.

Stokes, Donald and Stokes, Lillian. *Stokes Field Guide to Birds, Western Region*. Boston: Little, Brown & Co., 1996.

Whitney, Stephen. *A Sierra Club Naturalist's Guide to the Pacific Northwest*. San Francisco: Sierra Club Books, 1989.

Additional Reading

For more on the basics of doing hikes and other outdoor activities with children:

Cary, Alice. *Parents' Guide to Hiking & Camping: A Trailside Guide*. W.W. Norton & Co., 1997.

Doan, Marlyn. *The Sierra Club Family Outdoors Guide: Hiking, Backpacking, Camping, Bicycling, Water Sports and Winter Activities with Children*. San Francisco: Sierra Club Books, 1995.

Ross, Cindy and Gladfelter, Todd. *Kids in the Wild: A Family Guide to Outdoor Recreation*. Seattle: The Mountaineers, 1995.

Silverman, Goldie. *Backpacking with Babies and Small Children: A Guide to Taking the Kids Along on Day Hikes, Overnighters and Long Trail Trips*. Berkeley: Wilderness Press, 1998.

For general information on plants and animals:

The Peterson First Guides are excellent field guides for anyone learning about the natural world. There were 18 guides at last count, covering everything from astronomy to wildflowers. Some I'd recommend:

• *Peterson First Guide to Birds of North America*, Roger Tory Peterson, 1998
• *Peterson First Guide to Butterflies and Moths*, Paul Opler, 1998
• *Peterson First Guide to Forests*, John Kricher, 1999
• *Peterson First Guide to Insects of North America*, Roger Tory Peterson, 1998
• *Peterson First Guide to Mammals of North America*, Peter Alden and Roger Tory Peterson, 1998
• *Peterson First Guide to Reptiles and Amphibians*, Roger Conant et al., 1999
• *Peterson First Guide to Trees*, George Petrides and Roger Tory Peterson, 1998

For more information on British Columbia natural history:

Acorn, John and Sheldon, Ian. *Bugs of British Columbia*. Edmonton: Lone Pine Publishing, 2001.

Barwise, Joanne. *Animal Tracks of Western Canada*. Edmonton: Lone Pine Publishing, 1989.

Davis, James. *Seasonal Guide to the Natural Year: Oregon, Washington, British Columbia*. Golden, CO: Fulcrum Publishing, 1996.

Eder, Tamara. *Mammals of British Columbia*. Edmonton: Lone Pine Publishing, 2001.

Finlay, Joy and Cam, eds. *Ocean to Alpine: A British Columbia Nature Guide*. Edmonton: Lone Pine Publishing, 1992.

Hartson, Tamara. *Squirrels of the West*. Edmonton: Lone Pine Publishing, 1999.

Kavanagh, James. *Nature BC: An Illustrated Guide to Common Plants and Animals*. Edmonton: Lone Pine Publishing, 1993.

Kershaw, Linda, MacKinnon, Andy and Pojar, Jim. *Plants of the Rocky Mountains*. Edmonton: Lone Pine Publishing, 1998.

Lyons, C. P. and Merilees, Bill. *Trees, Shrubs and Flowers to Know in British Columbia and Washington*. Vancouver: Lone Pine Publishing, 1995.

MacKinnon, Andy, Pojar, Jim and Coupé, Ray. *Plants of Northern British Columbia*. Vancouver: Lone Pine Publishing, 1992.

Parish, Roberta, Coupé, Ray and Lloyd, Dennis. *Plants of Southern Interior British Columbia*. Vancouver: Lone Pine Publishing, 1996.

Sheldon, Ian. *Seashore of British Columbia*. Edmonton: Lone Pine Publishing, 1998.

Vitt, Dale, Marsh, Janet and Bovey, Robin. *Mosses, Lichens and Ferns of Northwest North America*. Edmonton: Lone Pine Publishing, 1988.

Wareham, Bill, Whyte, Gary and Kennedy, Shane. *British Columbia Wildlife Viewing Guide*. Edmonton: Lone Pine Publishing, 1991.

Information Sources

Maps or Other Trail Information

For the following regional parks, call the Greater Vancouver Regional District Parks Department at (604) 432-6350: Belcarra, Boundary Bay, Burnaby Lake, Campbell Valley, Capilano River, Crippen (Bowen Island), Deas Island, Derby Reach, Iona Beach, Kanaka Creek, Lynn Headwaters, Minnekhada, Pacific Spirit, Tynehead and Widgeon Marsh.

Alice Lake Provincial Park: BC Parks' Garibaldi Office, 1 (604) 898-3678
Blackie Spit: Surrey Parks Department, (604) 501-5050
Brandywine Provincial Park: BC Parks' Garibaldi Office, 1 (604) 898-3678
Burnaby Mountain Park: Burnaby Parks Department, (604) 294-7450
Cougar Mountain: BC Forest Service, Squamish District, 1 (604) 898-2100
Cypress Falls: West Vancouver Parks Department, (604) 925-7200
Cypress Provincial Park: BC Parks' Lower Mainland District Office, (604) 463-3513
Delta Nature Reserve: Burns Bog Conservation Society, (604) 572-0373
Fraser Foreshore Park: Burnaby Parks Department, (604) 294-7450
George C. Reifel Migratory Bird Sanctuary: (604) 946-6980
Golden Ears Provincial Park: BC Parks' Lower Mainland District Office, (604) 463-3513
Jericho Park: Vancouver Parks Board, (604) 257-8400
Lighthouse Park: West Vancouver Parks Department, (604) 925-7200
Lost Lake Park and trails: Resort Municipality of Whistler, 1 (604) 935-8104
Lynn Canyon Park: North Vancouver District Parks Department, (604) 990-3800, or the Ecology Centre, (604) 981-3103
Maplewood Flats Conservation Area: Wild Bird Trust, (604) 924-2581
Mount Seymour Provincial Park: BC Parks' Lower Mainland District Office, (604) 924-2200
Mundy Park: Coquitlam Parks Department, (604) 927-3530
Redwood Park: Surrey Parks Department, (604) 501-5050
Richmond Nature Park: (604) 718-6188
Serpentine Fen Wildlife Management Area and Pitt Wildlife Management Area: BC Ministry of Water, Land and Air Protection, (604) 582-5200
Seymour Demonstration Forest: (604) 987-1273
Shoreline Park: Port Moody Parks Department, (604) 469-4555
Squamish Estuary: Squamish Estuary Conservation Society, Box 1274, Squamish, BC, V0N 3G0
Stanley Park: Vancouver Parks Board, (604) 257-8400
UBC Research Forest: (604) 463-8148

Transportation

Ayla Canoe Rentals: (604) 941-2822, e-mail <rental@aylacanoes.com>, website <http://www.aylacanoes.com>
BC Ferries: 1-888-BCFERRY (1-888-223-3779), website <www. bcferries.bc.ca>
TransLink (city bus information): (604) 453-4500, website <www.translink.bc.ca>

Clothing & Equipment

Kids Outdoor Clothing

The following stores sell new outdoor kids clothing:
Altus: 137 West Broadway, Vancouver, (604) 876-5255
Coast Mountain: 2201 West Fourth, Vancouver, (604) 731-6181
Mountain Equipment Co-op: 130 West Broadway, Vancouver, (604) 872-7858, <www.mec.ca>
You can also sometimes find used outdoor clothing for kids at consignment stores. (It's a good idea to call first to see if the store has much outdoor stuff in stock.)

Baby Carriers

There are many baby carriers on the market. The best that I've found is the Baby Trekker designed and developed by a mom from Flin Flon, Manitoba. You can find Baby Trekkers in the Lower Mainland at the following stores:

Boomers & Echoes: 1709 Lonsdale, North Vancouver, (604) 984-6163
Camelot Kids: Kids Only Market, Granville Island, (604) 688-9766
Kuddel Muddel: 4342 Gallant, North Vancouver, (604) 929-2524
Room for Two Maternity: 1409 Commercial, Vancouver, (604) 255-0508
Soothers Boutique: 935 Marine Drive, North Vancouver, (604) 980-7229

You can find more information on the Baby Trekker at <www.babytrekker.com>. The company also offers mail order, but only if you're in an area where no stores retail the Baby Trekker.

If you can't stretch your budget for a new Baby Trekker, check the kids consignment stores. You may not find a Baby Trekker, but you might find a carrier that is in good repair with good support and padding. Call first to see if the store has any used baby carriers in stock.

Baby Backpacks

The following stores sell new baby backpacks:
A.J. Brooks: 147 West Broadway, Vancouver, (604) 874-1117, <www.ajbrooks.com>
Altus: 137 West Broadway, Vancouver, (604) 876-5255
Coast Mountain: 2201 West Fourth, Vancouver, (604) 731-6181
Europe Bound: 195 West Broadway, Vancouver, (604) 874-7456
Mountain Equipment Co-op: 130 West Broadway, Vancouver, (604) 872-7858, <www.mec.ca>
Taiga: 390 West Eighth, Vancouver, (604) 875-6644
TJ's The Kiddies Store: 3331 Jacombs, Richmond, (604) 270-8830, <www.tjskids.com>
Three Vets: 2200 Yukon, Vancouver, (604) 872-5475
Valhalla Pure: 222 West Broadway, Vancouver, (604) 872-8872

Occasionally, you can find second-hand baby backpacks at kids or sports consignment stores. The following are your best bets:
Cheapskates: 3496 Dunbar, (604) 734-1191
Sports Junkies: 600 West Sixth, Vancouver, (604) 879-0666 and 3056 St. Johns, Port Moody, (604) 469-3700

For a used backpack, the Baby Center website has an easily searchable recall section at <http://www.babycenter.com/safety#recall>.

All-terrain Strollers

Most bike stores sell all-terrain strollers. You can also find them at some kids equipment stores and running stores. Some that you can try include the following:
Reckless Bike Store: 1810 Fir, Vancouver, (604) 731-2420
Running Room: eight locations in the Lower Mainland; check the white pages or <www.runningroom.com>
Simon's Bike Shop: 608 Robson, Vancouver, (604) 602-1181, <www.simonsbikeshop.com>
TJ's The Kiddies Store: 3331 Jacombs, Richmond, (604) 270-8830, <www.tjskids.com>

Rarely, you may be able to find second-hand all-terrain strollers at a kids or sports consignment store. You may have better luck scanning the classified ads in such publications as Buy & Sell. There's an online version at <www.buysell.com>. Look under 'Children's and Nursery Furniture and Accessories.'

Hikes by Duration

1 to 1.5 hours

Brackendale Dykes
Maplewood Flats
Redwood Park
Yew Lake

1.5 to 2 hours

Goldie and Flower Lakes
Jericho Park
Kanaka Creek
Lighthouse Park
Lynn Canyon
Minnekhada
Reifel Migratory Bird Sanctuary
Tynehead Regional Park
UBC Malcolm Knapp
    Research Forest

2 to 2.5 hours

Admiralty Point
Alice Lake
Blackie Spit
Boundary Bay
Brandywine Falls
Brunswick Point
Burnaby Lake
Burnaby Mountain
Burns Bog (Delta Nature
    Reserve)
Campbell Valley
Capilano Canyon

Colony Farm
Cypress Falls
Deas Island
Derby Reach
Fraser Foreshore
Grey Rock
Hollyburn Ridge
Iona Beach
Killarney Lake
Lost Lake
Lower Seymour Conservation
    Reserve
Mundy Lake
Richmond Nature Park
Serpentine Fen
Shoreline Park
Squamish Estuary
Stanley Park
Towers Beach

2.5 to 3 hours

Cougar Mountain
Dog Mountain
Gold Creek Falls
Lynn Headwaters
Pacific Spirit Park South
Pitt Wildlife Marsh
Rainbow Falls
Widgeon Falls
    (plus paddling time)

Hikes by Difficulty

Easy
Blackie Spit
Boundary Bay
Brackendale Dykes
Brandywine Falls
Brunswick Point
Burnaby Lake
Burns Bog (Delta Nature
  Reserve)
Campbell Valley
Colony Farm
Deas Island
Fraser Foreshore
Iona Beach
Jericho Park
Killarney Lake
Lost Lake
Maplewood Flats
Minnekhada
Mundy Lake
Pacific Spirit Park South
Redwood Park
Reifel Migratory Bird Sanctuary
Richmond Nature Park
Serpentine Fen
Shoreline Park
Squamish Estuary
Stanley Park
Towers Beach
Tynehead Regional Park
Yew Lake

Easy to Moderate
Admiralty Point
UBC Malcolm Knapp
  Research Forest

Moderate
Alice Lake
Burnaby Mountain
Capilano Canyon
Cougar Mountain
Cypress Falls
Derby Reach
Dog Mountain
Gold Creek Falls
Goldie and Flower Lakes
Hollyburn Ridge
Kanaka Creek
Lighthouse Park
Lower Seymour Conservation
  Reserve
Lynn Canyon
Lynn Headwaters
Pitt Wildlife Marsh
Widgeon Falls

Tough
Grey Rock
Rainbow Falls

Hikes by Season

Year-round
Admiralty Point
Alice Lake
Blackie Spit
Boundary Bay
Brackendale Dykes
Brunswick Point
Burnaby Lake
Burnaby Mountain
Burns Bog (Delta Nature
    Reserve)
Campbell Valley
Capilano Canyon
Colony Farm
Cypress Falls
Deas Island
Derby Reach
Fraser Foreshore
Gold Creek Falls
Grey Rock
Iona Beach
Jericho Park
Kanaka Creek
Killarney Lake
Lighthouse Park
Lower Seymour Conservation
    Reserve
Lynn Canyon
Lynn Headwaters
Maplewood Flats
Minnekhada
Mundy Lake
Pacific Spirit Park South
Pitt Wildlife Marsh
Redwood Park
Reifel Migratory Bird Sanctuary
Richmond Nature Park
Serpentine Fen
Shoreline Park
Squamish Estuary
Stanley Park
Tynehead Regional Park
UBC Malcolm Knapp Research
    Forest
Widgeon Falls

May to October
Brandywine Falls
Cougar Mountain
Lost Lake
Rainbow Falls

June to October
Dog Mountain
Hollyburn Ridge
Yew Lake

July to September
Goldie and Flower Lakes

October to April
Towers Beach

Index to the Hikes

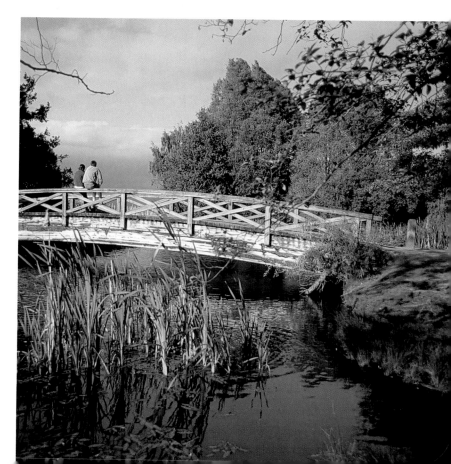

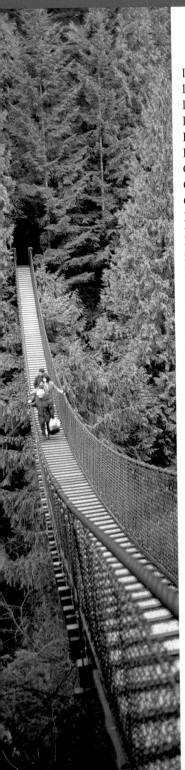

About the Author

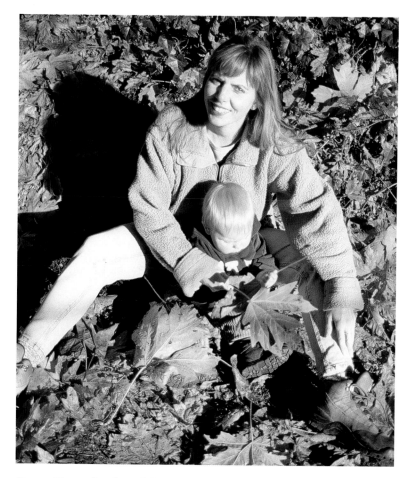

Dawn Hanna has been hiking since she was a young girl. With her family, she explored the trails of Capilano Canyon, Lighthouse Park, Mount Seymour and other places in the Lower Mainland.

As an adult, she has hiked throughout Canada, the United States and abroad, including such places as Chile, Argentina, Spain, Scotland and Mexico. Now, as a first-time mom, she is introducing another generation of family to the trails.

Dawn is the author of the best-selling *Best Hikes and Walks of Southwestern British Columbia.* She is the hiking columnist for the Adventure! section in *The Province* and has also written outdoor articles for such publications as *Beautiful British Columbia, The Georgia Straight, The Globe and Mail* and *Homemaker's.*

British Columbia...Outside Your Door

BEST HIKES AND WALKS OF SOUTHWESTERN BRITISH COLUMBIA
by Dawn Hanna

Author and well-known journalist Dawn Hanna covers the spectacular hikes to be experienced within about three hours of Vancouver. Notes on natural history and aboriginal lore are combined with important hiking information.

Softcover • 4.25" x 8.25" • 360 pages • ISBN 1-55105-095-1 • $19.95

MAMMALS OF BRITISH COLUMBIA
by Tamara Eder and Don Pattie

Identify and learn about 125 terrestrial and marine mammals of British Columbia with this colourful field guide. Detailed physical descriptions of the mammals accompany fascinating life history information. Includes tracks and up-to-date range maps, along with colour photographs and illustrations.

Softcover • 5.5" x 8.5" • 296 pages • ISBN 1-55105-299-7 • $26.95

WHALES AND OTHER MARINE MAMMALS OF BRITISH COLUMBIA AND ALASKA
by Tamara Eder
illustrated by Ian Sheldon

Whether you venture out on the high seas or observe nature from the shore, you'll enjoy this full-colour guide to the whales, dolphins, seals, sea-lions and other aquatic mammals of the Pacific coast. Includes a quick reference guide, tips for spotting whales, sections on whale myths, whaling, evolution, biology and behaviour.

Softcover • 5.5" x 8.5" • 160 pages • ISBN 1-55105-268-7 • $16.95

BIRDS OF COASTAL BRITISH COLUMBIA
by Nancy Baron and John Acorn

Award-winning author Nancy Barron and Nature Nut John Acorn have teamed up to write this insightful book, complete with beautiful full-colour illustrations. More than 200 species of common West Coast birds are grouped by their similarity of appearance and colour-coded for quick identification.

Softcover • 5.5" x 8.5" • 240 pages • ISBN 1-55105-098-6 • $19.95

BUGS OF BRITISH COLUMBIA
by John Acorn and Ian Sheldon

Author and avid bugster John Acorn provides humorous and accessible accounts of 125 of the coolest bugs found in British Columbia, while Ian Sheldon's stunning colour illustrations bring each species to life.

Softcover • 5.5" x 8.5" • 160 pages • ISBN 1-55105-231-8 • $14.95

These and other books on British Columbia's great outdoors are available at your local bookseller, or order direct from Lone Pine Publishing at 1-800-661-9017.